10 INDELIBLES

Formidable Distinctive Individuals

selkirk4books
(P.A.Brown)

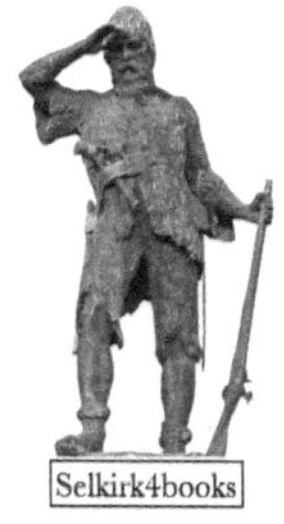

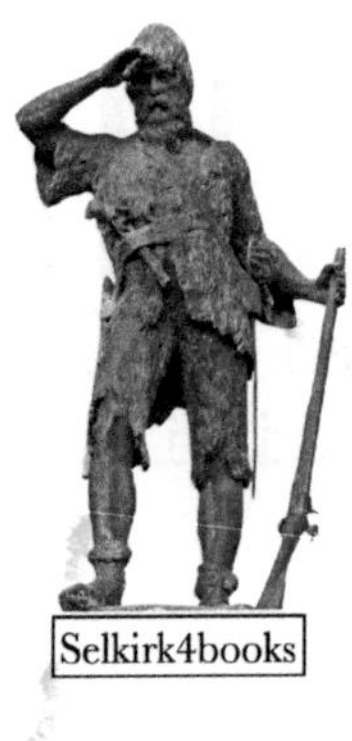

Copyright © 2023 Selkirk4books (P.A.Brown)

Updated 2025

All rights reserved The characters and events portrayed in this book are all genuine. No part of this book may be reproduced, or stored in a retrieval system, or transmitted in any form or by any means, electronic, mechanical, photocopying, recording, or otherwise, without express written permission of the publisher or author.

The author receives no commission from any of the links in this book.

Cover design by germancreative.

To my wife, TC, who in many ways
should have a chapter all her own.

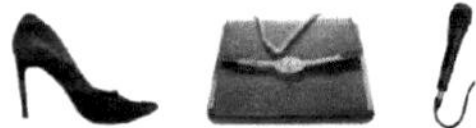

Contents

Introduction

How are you influenced? Do you consciously make decisions to stop being influenced by certain people, or do you just put up with the dislike, negativity, aggravation or annoyance of certain people, wishing you had the courage to do something about it? Conversely, have you ever gone out of your way to become involved with people who seem to live in a different world to yours? Most of us would say yes to both these.

As individuals, we are the sum of our interactions with the environment and people around us. Yet we rarely seem to find time to reflect on how others affect us—for good or bad.

Take an extreme example to bring home the point. Somewhere near mid-19thC Britain, a children's home was the scene of an experiment to discover what happens to babies without any stimuli. They were placed in white-sheeted cots, in a white-walled room with no stimuli of sounds, music, human voices or visual stimuli like mobiles, pictures or toys. Today, no-one would be surprised to learn that those babies died, even though adequately fed.

Another well-known example of the effects of isolation was ordered by Frederick II in 13thC Germany. The aim was to discover which language the children would develop into speaking if never spoken to. Of course, in those days there was much superstitious nonsense, which at that time validated their experiment. They fully expected the infants would end up speaking German! Yeah! Right!

Interestingly and unfortunately, another rule was imposed. The nurses were not allowed to touch the infants—taken from their mothers at birth. One wonders how the babies' nappies were changed!

The result of the experiment was not at all what Frederick and his team expected, though no-one today would be surprised to hear all the babies died.

So there is no argument that we all develop through contact with our immediate family and those others seen and heard in the routine of normal daily life.

What about the attempts to increase a child's IQ? (Bearing in mind this is only one way of measuring a child's potential).

Einstein was once questioned by a mother of a young primary school-aged child, *"What is the best thing to do to improve my child's intelligence?"*

"Read fairy stories to him." The mother was impatient with such an unexpected answer. So she added, *"Well, what is the second best thing?"*

"Read more fairy stories to him."

Slightly irritated by now, she asked, *"OK, but what would be your third point?"*

"Read even more fairy stories to him," he said.

In other words, he was telling the mother to stimulate the child's imagination, rather than try to fill his head with facts.

Now, consider this. In remote villages in places with no external stimuli like TV, internet, books, or travellers mingling with the villagers—what would be the likely intellectual and world-view capacity of the villagers?

Historically, this was the situation for millions of isolated villages and towns around the world. New things divulged by strangers suddenly appearing in your village or town would be instantly regarded with fear and suspicion, though change, albeit slowly, was inevitable.

Another way of changing the way a person is developing may be a sudden or emerging determination to resolve a situation you find yourself in. A good example is Arnold Schwarzenegger, as a teenager, being fronted close up, face to face with his father snarling the words, *"You'll never amount to anything."*

So, excusing this laboured description, it can be said that as individuals, our world view or philosophy of life, and character too, is determined by the level of one's life experiences starting at birth. For me, this book's ten people influenced me in more powerful ways than the usual run-of-the-mill life experiences. They immeasurably changed me.

I have deliberately avoided the mention of DNA though mention is needed of one sobering fact (as far as science is currently able to judge). It is that only about 10% of our inherited genes affect our lives, including mental and physical health, and disease.

So, lifestyle, which involves our interactions with other people, accounts for the way we are. However, a necessary waiver is the so far unexplained brilliance in some infants and young children that appears to come from nowhere. A current example is of a 24 month old boy living in a village south of Saigon, Vietnam. The parents work in the local factory, and neither has any further-education qualifications.

While watching TV with her son, the mother was astounded to hear her little boy read the words appearing on the screen. It turned out he could read English and Vietnamese without ever having been taught. There is no rational explanation, to date, about how this appearance of great skills can happen. Thanks to the internet, these 'instant geniuses' or child prodigies are now seen to be more common than expected. Savants, too, are those who have exceptional aptitude, usually in one particular area, like mathematics, languages, etc. Many are handicapped; think 'Rain Man', the movie, about an autistic savant.

This brings me to the point of this book. Travelling widely, I have met people living in a variety of cultures. I have engaged in long conversations with them, lived with them for a while, and sometimes worked with them. Now, looking back over the years, I realise there are some significant stand-out people who radically changed my thinking and belief system—my world view of life.

They were influential towards me in different ways. They have indelibly affected the way I think and live. Importantly, this has provided me with a high level of satisfaction in living more calmly, simply and without envy or jealousy of other people's assets. So they have become my indelibles.

Of the people I write about, the apparent gender bias is unintended. Perhaps a female writing this book would have a higher number of females?

Chapter One

SWEIN MACDONALD

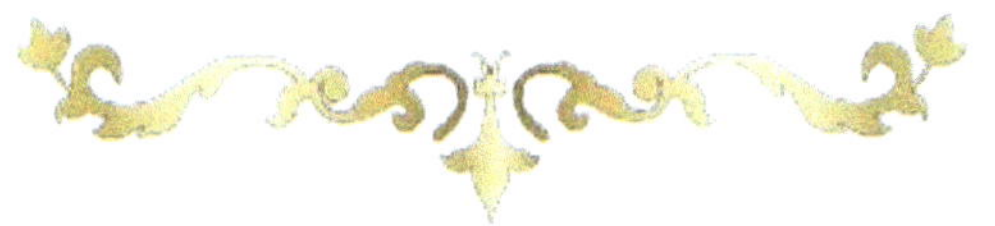

Highland Seer

(1931-2003)

"The seer sees." — Lailah Gifty Akita

When we hear the word 'seer' we usually think of historical characters like Nostradamus, Edgar Cayce, Old Mother Shipton, Elizabeth Barton, Baba Vanga, Emanuel Swedenborg and Alois Irlmaier to name a few.

In the Highlands of Scotland there is a level of pride in the 17th Century Brahan Seer, known in Scottish Gaelic as Coinneach Odhar. Although there is no firm historical evidence that he ever existed, it is possible, even probable, historians have confused elements of passed-down prophesies and actual records. An outstanding example from 16th Century records is of a Coinneach Odhar who was accused of witchcraft. Whatever the truth is, the predictions were astonishing.

When I went with my young family to live on the Isle of Skye in the 1970's, I was learning as much as I could about the Highlands. I was appalled how my learned English history, while a student in England, compared to the history as taught to Highland children. Basically, my English version omitted the horrors committed by the English towards the Highlanders.

It was while reading a magazine article I first heard about the Brahan Seer who used an Adder stone, a stone with a hole through its middle, to see into the future. Then the article mischievously talked about the current Brahan Seer, a man called Swein Macdonald. It was many years later before I found out that he had named himself the Highland Seer and didn't associate himself with the historical Brahan Seer. However, many people do, though by association rather than attributable facts.

I was still intrigued by what I read about Swein, for he had predicted many astonishing things. One of his most quoted happened years after reading the article. A few days before it happened, he predicted the Braer Disaster off Shetland in 1993. The MV Braer tanker ran aground in a Force 11 gale on the southern tip of Shetland and spilled twice as much crude oil as the Exxon Valdez, which ran aground off Alaska four years previously. Most people recall the latter because there was far more media coverage of that disaster.

I looked up Swein's name in the telephone directory and gave him a call. What followed was nothing short of astonishing. I introduced myself by saying I had very recently moved from England to the Isle of Skye and read an article about him. Without any pleasantries at all, he said, *"You are shortly being visited by three, blonde-haired children."*

I confirmed this fact while at the same time wondering how on earth a man I had never met before could know this. My ex-wife's three children from an earlier marriage were indeed arriving on their school summer holidays within a few more days. Swein then launched into the following. *"You have a lean-to shed on the side of your house that you use as a work shop."*

With incredulity, I said, *" Yes."*

Without pause he continued, *"On the bench I see a circular saw blade without a safety cover. The teeth are sticking up."*

I was speechless. I was in the process of building a powered circular saw. I had reached the stage of being ready to connect the under-bench motor. I had not yet found a cover for the saw teeth.

Swein went on, *"One of those children, the younger boy, will climb up on the bench to reach a tool hanging from the roof."*

Yes, there were quite a few tools hanging over the bench from hooks on the timber frame of the tin roof. And he seemed to know that there were two boys and one girl from the language he had just used.

"Either remove the saw or cover it well, as the boy will fall on the saw if you don't."

I thanked him, saying I'd remove the saw blade right away. Three days later the children arrived and enjoyed playing with my own two young children. There were goats, horses, sheep, chickens, a dog and a cat to keep them interested and busy. Then one morning, I went out of the back door to the lean-to shed. Just as I arrived at the open door there was a cry and a thud. I saw Jonathon sprawled over the edge of the bench, exactly where the circular saw blade had been before I removed it. He said he was trying to reach a tool he wanted. The same thought repeatedly crossed my mind. If I hadn't have made that call to Swein, Jonathon would have been injured, possibly seriously.

Naturally, I started taking much more interest in this seer business though research was a hard slog before the internet. I became interested in the 7th son of a 7th son in respect of healing powers, prophecies and second sight. For centuries in Europe and USA it has been believed that the 7th son of a 7th son is endowed with prophetic vision (second sight) and occult powers. Often they have healing powers too.

This belief in occult powers of a 7th son of a 7th son, or daughter, persists into the twenty first century[1]. Swein MacDonald was born in Nairn on the seventh day of the seventh month, a date of astral significance though not quite the same thing as a 7th son, or a 7th son of a 7th son. The biblical David may have been a 7th son, though there are conflicting references about that in the bible.

I wanted to meet Swein. I arranged an appointment through his wife Isabelle. It was a 3 hour drive across northern Scotland from my then home on Skye to his cottage in Ardgay, at the head of the Dornoch Firth on the east side of northern Scotland. I was met with a firm handshake from this bearded, roughly dressed seer. He withdrew his hand abruptly and muttered something.

"What?" I asked, hesitatingly.

"Hard life, hard life," is all he said, very quietly.

This I reflect on now and again when I look back on my life, and wonder what else may come.

He took us in and offered us tea. His long suffering wife soon brought in a tray of refreshments. I say long suffering not unkindly, but because she was credited as having as good a gift of prediction as Swein but allowed him first place, so to speak, by becoming his secretary and arranging appointments.

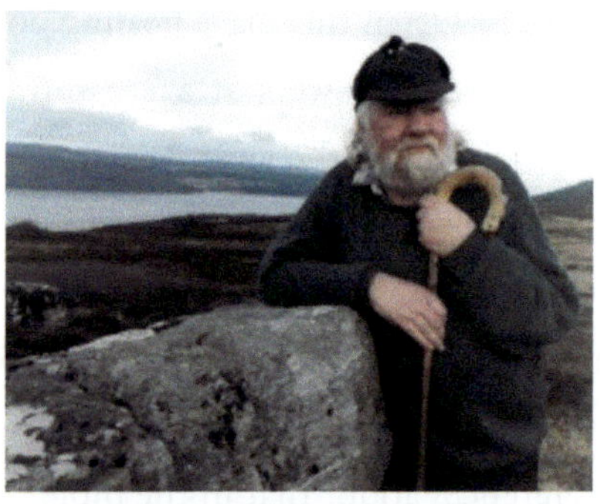

Swein Macdonald at home.
Image courtesy Barbara Meiklejohn-Free
The Highland Seer

In Swein's own words he describes how he interviewed his clients: *"It's like watching a slow-moving film. As we talk, I begin to see images rolling along, instances from their past, people they know and what happened to them; sometimes the film quickens and I have to rush to get things out, then it slows down again. But if I see something black or tragic in the future, I refrain from telling people. I am not in the business of frightening folk."*

I visited him in the mid-seventies. His way of interviewing, as described above, fitted well with how he talked with me. He described seeing marching soldiers, in his sitting room. He had pointed at an angle, down towards one side of the room as he spoke. He said the soldiers were of long ago, before his cottage was built.

I asked when was it he realised he had these special attributes. He surprised me by saying that working as an engineer on a building site, a crane hook swung and hit him hard on the back of his head. This caused tunnel vision. From that point on it all started. That's what he told me, person to person, though there is an account that tells he was a stonemason and he gave up the work when bricks fell on his head, nearly killing him. There are other accounts that agree with what he personally told me.

I then talked about the reason I wanted to see him. My family and I were soon going to emigrate to Australia. We were required to have a sponsor already living there. My brother had a good friend whose older brother had emigrated to Queensland years ago. I'd contacted him and he was willing to sponsor us on the condition I worked for him. My ex wife had a very distant relative who'd emigrated to Western Australia many years ago. I'd written to him also and he'd agreed to sponsor us if I worked for him. Choosing between these two sponsors seemed to be a simple case of opting for our preferred part of Australia and its climate.

Sitting next to Swein I produced the two letters. My intention was to take out the letters from their envelopes and let him read them to see if his prophetic skills would shed some light on my family's future. He held out his hand and took them as they were, in their envelopes. He said he didn't need to read them, just hold them. With one in each hand, he closed his eyes. His hands moved a little as they held the envelopes.

On opening his eyes, he said, *"This one is a kind, honest and reasonable man. He would be a good boss."*

Looking at the other envelope, he went on, *"This man is a slave-driver and will work you into the ground."*

I took the envelopes from him, carefully making sure I would remember which was which by marking the better one with an asterisk. After thanking him and his wife we left for the long drive back home.

The talk, naturally, was about choosing the sponsor in Western Australia — the good boss, and wondering how we would like WA.

***

Nearly a year later the family was finally able to set off for Western Australia. We thought we were lucky because Western Australia is well known for its beautiful Mediterranean climate.

It's funny how things can turn out. Two days after our arrival I was working 12 hour-shifts, 6 days a week while the rest of the family explored their new city and enjoyed the beaches. More than once I wondered if Swein had got it right!

It was only after some months when we were able to move into a house of our own and reorganise our things, that the two letters surfaced among lots of other papers and documents.

Imagine the disbelief on discovering the two letters, from the very beginning, had not been returned to their correct envelopes. This meant that the kind boss lived in Queensland, not Western Australia! Well, I suppose at least we had avoided the east coast humidity!

Sadly, Swein passed away in 2003[2].

REFERENCES/LINKS

[1] Search: "7th sons" There are many references.

[2] Search: "BBC archive video of Swein Macdonald"

Many articles about Swein. Search: "Swein Macdonald"

CHAPTER TWO

JOHN TONKIN

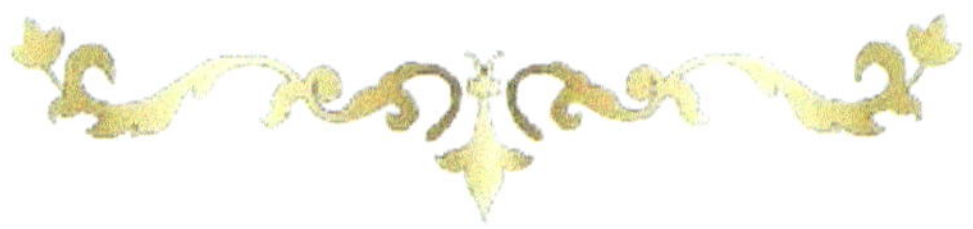

THE EYES HAVE IT

(1902-1993)

"Marilla is eighty-five," said Anne with a sigh. "Her hair is snow-white. But, strange to say, her eyesight is better than it was when she was sixty." — L.M. Montgomery

John Tonkin[1], the 20th Premier of Western Australia, was known as "Honest John". An unusual nickname for a politician, it has to be said. He had another unusual personal characteristic that few people seem aware of.

Around 1988 I read a newspaper article about him that mentioned he had 20-20 vision, even at his advanced age. I was immediately interested to read the whole article because I had always wanted to confirm my belief that glasses ought to be unnecessary if we do the right things. I searched the telephone directory for his number, and found the page for the state government. I wasn't very hopeful. I tried a number and amazingly, was speaking to him directly. His first words were, "How did you get this number?"

Somehow, I had got lucky! I don't think it was meant to be that easy! Perhaps it was a dysfunctional automatic redirection.

I explained why I was trying to contact him and as soon as I mentioned eye sight, he was happy to chat. I later met him in the Government House Gardens in Perth at the John Tonkin Tree Awards in 1990, where my students were the winners of the Certificate of Merit.

A couple of decades earlier I had read about an American Ophthalmic Optician called William Bates who accidentally discovered a way of being able to discard his own use of glasses. One day, he was particularly tired after seeing patients the whole morning, and retired to a quiet store room and sat with his elbows on his knees and his hands holding his head. His cupped hands covered his eyes and for a good 5 minutes he sat like that. When he stopped and stood up, he was surprised how his eyes reacted. He told how everything seemed much brighter than usual and colours were vivid. He believed having his eyes in darkness for a few minutes was responsible. He repeated this regularly and before long, threw away his own glasses.

There must be more to this than I have been able to find, but the Bates method has never scientifically been proven, though there are many anecdotal claims for improved eyesight by following his 'method'. In his explanations, Bates (1860 - 1931) insisted that the shape of the eyeball changes to accomodate focus by the action of the muscles surrounding the eyeballs. Although described by medics in that field of study as not proven, Bates was surely onto something, even if his explanation was scientifically inaccurate. He is still popular on the internet today.

The eyes have four main groups of muscles. The extra-ocular muscles control eye movement. There are six around each eye. Then there are the muscles of the iris whose function is to dilate and constrict the pupils, in other words control the amount of light entering the eyes. Then the eyelid muscles. Finally, the ciliary muscles, which surround the lens of each eye, have the function of changing the shape of the lens (not size of the pupil) to enable focusing on near and far details.

Now of these four groups of muscles, the extra-ocular and ciliary muscles are the ones that would, if not exercised enough, likely show most deterioration over time as one got older. This would obviously have an effect on the acuity of vision.

To me, this is the crux of the arguments and continual debates about so-called age-related eye problems. Should we expect to have to wear glasses as a result of ageing?

Diseases of the eye like cataracts, retinol disorders, conjunctivas, glaucoma and other optic nerve disorders have, to state the obvious, a reason for degeneration. The argument is whether growing older itself causes eye-related problems. I strenuously appose that viewpoint, which is anyway unsupported by research, though is eminently suitable for the financial success of the optician industry!

To digress a moment from John Tonkin and Bates, an example of where nutrition levels play a part in the health and acuity of the eyes and vision, is from a Queensland doctor who, in the 1980's, prescribed high Vit C doses for Aboriginal patients suffering glaucoma. Glaucoma appears to be quite common in Aboriginal people. His success with prescribing high doses of Vit C for glaucoma eventually got him noticed by the Australian Medical Association and a severe reprimand for prescribing it, as it is not recognised as the expected treatment from Australian doctors! A clear case, to me, of following medical rules being more important to the AMA than successful treatment.

Most unhealthy eye conditions, and other health conditions, stem from the effects of oxidation—which anyone with a functioning brain (apologies for the sarcasm) would realise is a direct consequence of one's diet, not age! If this were not so, then medical science needs to explain how some people, like John Tonkin, maintain 20/20 vision right to the end, over 90 years! So, having a poor diet, being diabetic, and/or having high levels of blood sugar and insulin, shout for an intake of antioxidant nutrients. Vit. E and Vit C. are great anti-oxidants yet almost always lacking in modern diets, certainly so with processed foods. They would very likely contribute to assisting eye health.

However, these two nutrients are not often mentioned because, as Dr Berg[2] in the USA points out, there is little research, strangely, about their connection to eye health. I know of one Queensland doctor who would raise his eyes at this! Getting back to John, he told me that since the age of 18, he maintained his quality of vision by exercising his eyes for 5 minutes on arising every morning. He told me of a conversation he had in Parliament with another politician.

"John, how is it possible, without glasses, you can read your notes when either holding your paperwork or looking down to your desk from a standing position?"

Rhetorically, John asked him if he had the wherewithal to do a five minute an exercise every morning, to which the reply was, *"Probably not!"*

Interestingly, of the eye muscles that may need exercising, John's exercise routine only included the extra-ocular muscles because his description to me was simply to stand upright and then, keeping the head still, look upwards as far as one can, pause, then downwards, pause, then sideways left, pause, then right, pause, then do circular movement of the eyes, clockwise and anticlockwise. Each time looking as far upwards, downwards, sideways and rotationally as is possible. Pushing the range of peripheral vision would be a good description. When first doing these exercises people experience soreness, just as happens when any muscle is suddenly made to start working again. This wears off after a few days of the exercise.

I have my own take on this. In days when people hunted prey, they would consciously use their peripheral vision much more and avoid movements of their head, which might alert the prey to the hunter's presence. In modern times, people always turn their head to see things directly in front of them. It would even be socially inappropriate to regard someone's presence out of the corner of one's eyes, instead of facing them directly. So the hunters exercised their peripheral vision while modern society doesn't.

Almost everyone's extra-ocular muscles lack a daily work-out, so, over the years, slowly atrophy. Some opticians have recommended standing at a window and alternatively focusing on a mark on the glass and then on a distant object, seen through the glass. This would exercise the ciliary muscles and is probably helpful, though John didn't do this.

Since talking to John, I have done his daily, 5 minutes eye exercises for over 30 years and while I know I haven't got 20-20 vision, I don't need glasses at my great age and can read books with a font size of 10 with ease, though I prefer 11. John Tonkin was living proof that his way works. Many people make health claims but rarely do we hear from people in their nineties, and perhaps even more rarely, about 20-20 vision!

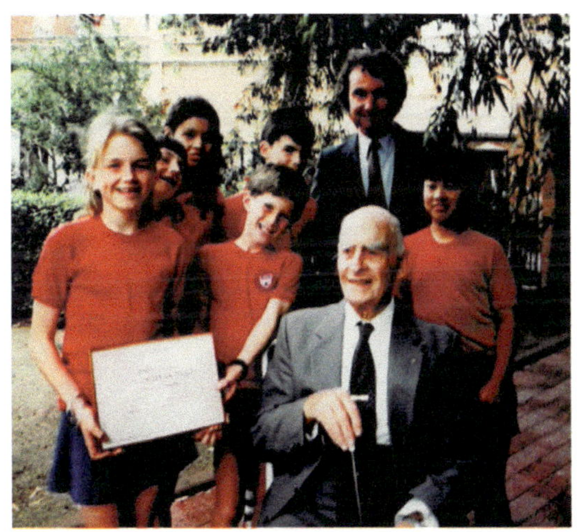

John Tonkin, seated, in Government House Gardens, Perth, Western Australia, for presentation of John Tonkin Tree Awards in 1990 to Students from Leederville Primary School
Image by author

Opticians appeal to those who think there is no alternative. The worst of this choice is that as soon as you wear glasses, you are facilitating the deterioration of your eye health and vision. Your glasses become a crutch. Then you will need to have repeated changes of glasses as time goes by, along with the not-inconsiderable expenses.

John passed away in 1995. John Tonkin will always get my vote!

REFERENCES/LINKS

[1] Born in 1902 in Boulder, Western Australia.

[2] Search: Dr *Berg eye health*

Many articles about John Tonkin: Search:

Tonkin Biography by J. Trezise

Chapter Three

DON GREENBANK

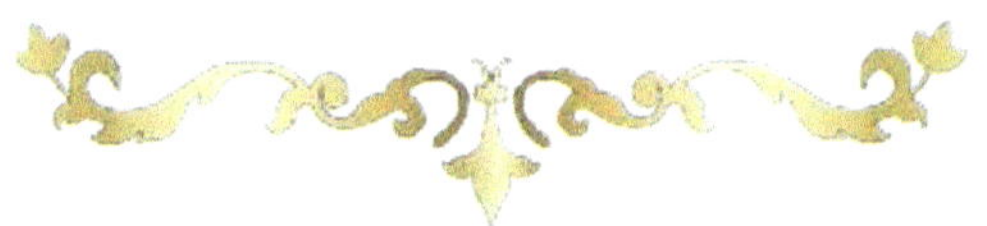

Phenomenal healer

(circa 1922-1992)

"Healing is an inside job." Dr B. J. Palmer

At 22 years old, I was trying to deal with an accidentally self-inflicted severe back problem. After 18 months of 24/7 severe pain and every intervention considered and tried—the final offer was surgery to fuse the lower vertebrae. I declined on instinct. It didn't feel right, especially at my age.

One day, while trying to get a little relief after work by lying flat on the sick-bed, a cleaning lady walked past, stopped, sighed, turned her head and said, *"You need to see Don."*

"Who's Don?" I asked.

"Oh, just go and see him."

She returned a minute later with the address scribbled on a piece of paper. I debated with myself as to whether I should bother. It was a cold, winter's day and all I wanted was to get home. I struggled into my vehicle and thought about it again. Finally I decided to at least go and see. My heart sank when I saw a street of old, dilapidated terraced houses. I pulled up outside and paused. Did I really want to bother. Was it going to be yet another pointless intervention or should I just go straight home and face another painful evening?

The fact of having arrived at the address made me decide to at least see what this was about. Slowly, with spasms of pain, I climbed out of the car. There was no signage or brass plate that might have given a clue as to what went on there. I knocked on the door and when no one answered, I tried the handle. It opened. I called out Hello. I could see a hall dresser with a donation box on it. That prompted me to open the door wider and step inside.

Still no one there but the atmosphere was palpable. So calm, peaceful and welcoming. I immediately felt comfortable and looked around the small hallway.

There was an open door on the left. I looked in and decided it must be a waiting room. I went in and slowly lowered myself into a comfortable, upholstered chair. I heard voices and the sound of someone leaving. Then a man looked in and asked me to follow him. I assumed this must be Don Greenbank, the person I had come to see. In this next room this so-far-predictable story became something hard to believe.

I saw a disproportionally large room. This puzzled me as these two-storey terraced houses were built exactly alike and are very small houses. In the centre of the room, all by itself, was an ordinary wooden dining chair. In the corner of the room nearest the door I'd just entered was an office area, to which Don went and sat for a moment shuffling papers. He said he would just be a moment. There was very quiet music playing which I later learned was Scheherazade. Then he stood up and said, as he walked towards me, *"Sit on the chair, sideways, please."*

Struggling, I took off my overcoat and he took it to the office corner and placed it on the edge of the desk. As he walked back I saw him scrutinising me. There was a suggestion of a smile on his face. I had started to take off my jacket but he said to leave it on, and just sit down. As I slowly sat down the door opened and in came a girl, probably in her early twenties. She was introduced as Karen.

On one knee, facing my left side, Don proceeded to place his hand on the middle of my back, just below my jacket collar. I started to tell him my problem but he interrupted and said it wasn't necessary. Maybe he'd decided my back was the problem from the way I walked in and carefully and slowly sat down. Anyway, he proceeded to slide his hand down my spine and then back to my collar. He repeated this twice and then stopped his hand on my lower back, exactly where I felt the most pain.

Karen, meanwhile, was standing facing me, and had placed her right palm on my forehead and the other on my left shoulder. I felt heat on my forehead from Karen's hand, and then noticed Don had started moving his hand in a circular motion over the sore area. Even through my layers of winter clothing, I felt warmth from his hand.

After only a couple of minutes, he stood up. Karen moved back a step.

Don said, *"OK, you're fixed. I want you to lean backwards and circle your body left and right."*

Remarkably the constant pain had stopped, but instinctively I grabbed the side of the chair with both hands, alarmed at the pain this would likely cause.

He smiled and said, *"Don't worry, I'll support you."*

Even so, I kept hold of the chair's back with my right hand while I tentatively leaned slowly backwards. No pain. I leaned further back. Still no pain. Don then helped me move in a circular movement, left and right, backwards and forwards. Still no pain. This was incredible. Gaining more confidence I started twisting my body backwards and left and right, reaching further than ever.

He asked me to stand. I did so and remarkably, still felt absolutely no pain. This was the first time there had been no pain in 18 months. I couldn't express my gratitude enough. I thanked them profusely and went to leave. To this day I regret walking past that donation box without even registering its presence, in spite of having noticed it earlier. I was totally preoccupied with feeling no pain whatsoever. Because Don was an untrained, unlicensed practitioner, the law forbad him to charge clients. So, a donation box was his only option. Years later he told me wealthy clients usually didn't donate and that poor people were the most generous. I was not exactly either, but regretfully had still failed to make a donation. I am writing this over 50 years after the event and still have no problems with my back. To science, this is just an anecdotal 'non-medical' intervention and so carries no weight. But for me, Don restored my life to normal and changed the way I thought about medical practice.

Now what I have just described may equate in your mind with many other instances of miraculous cures that go the rounds. That's as maybe, but what follows will leave you with an indelible wonder of Don.

Many years later Don Greenbank was living and working in a rather different house in the same city of Bradford, England. He had met his soulmate, Maggie. They lived in a grand, triple-glazed mansion on Greenbank Road — a hard-to-explain coincidence of names!

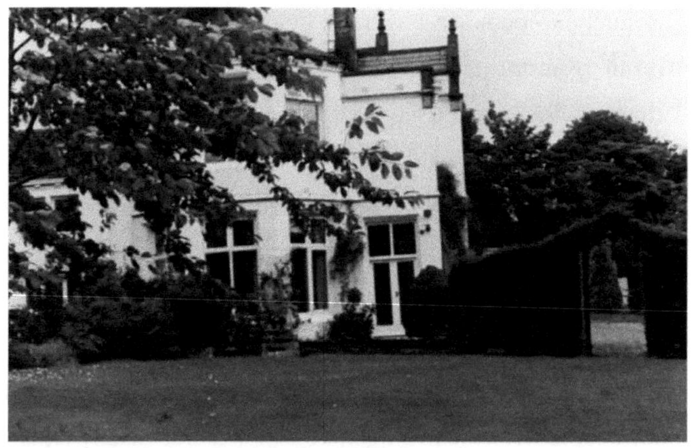

Don Greenbank's house in Greenbank Lane, Bradford, Yorkshire, England.
Image by author P.A.Brown

In his book, "A Healer's Pathway", is a long chapter called 'My Healing Mission to Israel'. He briefly describes his visits to Israel as the result of a patient who made a miraculous recovery, which led to 6 healing visits to that country. What he doesn't mention, probably due to political sensitivity at the time, is something he told me much later. A middle-aged female had come to his sanctuary, as he called his house and place of work, to be healed. She was completely cured and returned to London.

A few days later he had a call from the lady's husband. He asked if they might visit him. It turned out he was the Israeli Ambassador to Britain. He had been so overwhelmingly impressed with his wife's dramatic recovery that he invited Don to go to Israel to treat war victims, primarily, but also others. Don had hesitated slightly, wondering if he could afford to travel there and stay in a hotel and leave his sanctuary for an indeterminate number of weeks. The ambassador probably guessed the reason for Don's indecision and added that all his expenses would be covered. So Don went to Israel.

What Don recounted next was both hilarious and amazing. You see, over the years Don had developed a rather bad habit, it could be said, of having a sip of whisky after treating every patient. Now this was entirely his prerogative in a country like England, but not in a synagogue where alcohol is expressly forbidden! One fact I'm unsure of is which synagogue it was. Don described it to me as the main synagogue in Jerusalem. I have noticed through quick research that it was likely to be the Great Synagogue, consecrated by the Wolfson family in the memory of the six million Jews who perished in the Holocaust and to the fallen soldiers of Israel Defence Forces.

In any case, Don was shown into the synagogue and led to a table and chair on the ground floor, from where Don would heal people. Two things need to be realised at this point. Don, a Gentile (a non-Jew) is standing on the ground floor where only Jews are allowed. Gentiles can be present in the synagogue, but only upstairs in the balconies, not on the ground floor. The other thing only became evident to the rabbi and others there when Don put his little case on the table, opened it, and took out a bottle of whisky! There was a gasp of disbelief from all around. They admonished him for bringing alcohol inside but Don insisted that he needed the whisky to be able to heal. He said that it was his way of dealing with so many patients. Amazingly, they relented and so Don must be the only Gentile in history to have had permission to drink whisky on the ground floor of a synagogue.[1]

Don's visits to Israel were, to say the least, extremely successful and welcomed by all who saw or heard of Don, except, apparently, many GP doctors there who resented Don's amazing healing abilities.

After all-day healing sessions in the synagogue, he would return to the hotel looking forward to a long rest. However, every day when he returned to the hotel, there was a long queue of people waiting hopefully for a chance to meet this healer. Don told me the queue went all the way upstairs and along the corridor to his door. Word of mouth had been operating in advance of his arrival in Israel, apparently.

One healing described by Don in his book will illustrate how amazing his healing was:

"Possibly the quickest healing that happened in Israel took place within the space of a few seconds. Rabbi Yossi Rosenstine, probably best known the world over as a painter of Biblical scenes in the surrealist manner, brought his four year old son for healing. The child had been released from hospital that very morning suffering from what was termed an abscess of the lung, a diagnosis that had been confirmed several times previously by x-rays. I sat the little chap on my knee and having identified mentally where the trouble lay, sought healer's help for him. The healing energy that came for the little one was staggering in its intensity. It came like a bolt from heaven. Immediately I was told by my intuitive senses that the cure was full and complete. My words to the father were; 'All the pain has been removed. The abscess is now fully healed. Return to the hospital now and have further x-rays taken and the doctor will give you confirmation that the cure is complete.' The boy confirmed all the pain had gone. His breathing was normal, with none of the rasping sounds he had previously. With a smile of thankfulness the father dashed out with his son and returned within three hours, beaming all over his face. The x- rays and the doctor, had confirmed my words ... all to the utter consternation of the consultant who had examined him only hours earlier that very morning."[2]

I remember one dark winter's evening Don made his first visit to my house in East Morton, Yorkshire, England. There were no street lights outside, being in an unlit, hidden row of houses among trees alongside a stream in a little valley. When the knock on the door came, my Labrador went mad. I grasped her collar as I opened the door. There stood Don, smiling.

I said, *"Hang on. Let me put the dog in another room. She doesn't know you."*

"No, don't. Just watch," he said.

He bent forwards and downwards slightly, towards the now snarling, growling dog who needed a firm hand to hold her back. He put his hand out, palm foremost, towards her. She stopped snarling, relaxed her mouth and started to back away, turning her head left and right. Don told me to put my hand between his hand and the dog's face, a distance of about 75 cm. I felt an icy draft of air flowing towards the dog from Don's palm. How? I still have absolutely no idea, yet I felt it.

I miss Don. So too, I'm sure, will anyone who spent time with him. He frequently went hang gliding to relieve the stress of continuous healing. He was available to anyone 24/7. He introduced me to the sport. That feeling of flying like a bird, with the wind in your face, hundreds of feet high, is unlike anything else. I read of two jumbo jet pilots describing their joy at hang gliding, saying it was 'real flying'! Easy to see how Don was able to lose stress while flying like that. The following quote shows he was fun to be around:

"The late Don Greenbank was a very generous person. He would often let me fly his latest glider as a change from my old Argos. I remember an occasion at Addingham Floorside when he decided not to carry his bundled-up glider any further along the

ridge, involving 2 or 3 stiles. He took off not only forgetting to wear his helmet, but also that it was hanging from the outer end of the cross tube. His subsequent 360º at low level was a sight to see! There was never a dull moment when Don was around!" [3]

After moving to Australia in 1981 the contact with Don naturally diminished greatly. Emails and the internet hadn't started and Don wasn't the greatest letter writer. However, about 14 years later while travelling in South America, I had the opportunity of a so called 'free-leg flight' so long as the flight was backwards to the direction of travel around the world for the ticket I had purchased. I was able to travel from Chile to UK and back to Chile, free of charge.

I had a list of people to visit and Don was one of the first. I still remember the moment I rang the doorbell and heard him shout to come in. I went through to the doorway of a large room. He was standing with his back to the large fireplace, on the opposite side of the room, with one elbow resting on the mantlepiece.

He said, *"Let me have a look - oh no, your left shoulder is down again!"*

I started to walk towards him, knowing that he would 'adjust' my shoulder back to a more optimal position, as he had done a few times before. He told me to stop, and just stand where I was.

From across the room, at a distance of 6-7 metres, he started telling me he had moved away from 'hands-on' healing and now used remote healing. This was the first I had heard of this! I actually felt pressure on my back and shoulder and thought someone must have crept up quietly behind me and started manipulating my shoulder. I turned to see who it was, and Don laughed, then said, *"OK that's better now. Your shoulders are level."* He said that people found it hard to believe how he could treat anyone without his former 'hands-on' approach. It does defy common sense!

A couple of other things have come to mind since writing the above. Don told me that a few times, sometimes once a week, after a full day of healing, he would find a thick layer of hard, whitish, grease-like substance over the soles of his feet. He never did find out exactly what it was, but assumed it was his body's way of dealing with stress. He had to scrape it off!

Another thing he told me was how regularly, every week, he would get pensioners, usually female, coming to see him alone or in pairs. They would not have anything significantly or obviously wrong with them. They just enjoyed the attention from being with Don and walked out feeling so much better. For Don, they unfortunately represented a big drain on his energy levels.

Once, he told me that his sanctuary in the terraced house I had first visited, was such a quiet and peaceful place to be, but only on the ground floor. He felt uneasy if he ever went upstairs and so, rarely did. Also, he said once, while healing in the large room where he fixed my back, he saw a face at the only window of the room. What was unusual about this is that there was no entry to the little area at the back, only through the window itself. There were other houses sealing off the small area between them.

That Don endured stress was not immediately obvious to people. If he knew you well, he would occasionally talk about it. He told me that hang-gliding was his way of losing stress. He described how once he went with a group of hang-gliders to Robin Hood's Bay on the Yorkshire coast. He decided to have a flight from some cliffs the group was walking past. The updraft of wind at a cliff face usually guarantees an interesting flight. He was the only one who wanted to take off from that particular place, so the others just watched. He took off over the cliff and was quickly lifted upwards to about 200 feet, but was caught in what was called 'a curl-over', caused by a sudden squall of snow and gale force wind. This in turn inverted the hang-glider wing through the sudden down-pressure. He was slammed into the ground from this great height.

His friends rushed to help him. He was groaning and complained of having hurt his back. With immense relief he was able to wiggle his toes and fingers. As he lay on the ground he noticed soccer goalposts reasonably close by and asked his flying friends to help him over to them. He got them to hold him up high enough for him to grasp the top bar, and then asked them to pull downwards on his legs. His thinking was to stretch out his spine. As luck would have it, the top bar snapped in half and he was back groaning on the ground again!

His friends drove him home and carried him to bed. Even the slightest movement sent spasms of pain throughout his body. Even so he was thinking of his hundreds of patients booked in for healing. He refused to go to hospital, knowing they would impose complete bed rest for weeks. Instead he had some friends take him to his sanctuary where he treated patients from a borrowed wheelchair.

In his words, *"I made the lovely discovery that while I was treating people I had no pain at all."* By sheer determination he carried on healing from a wheelchair for the six weeks it took for his spine to normalise.

Another account he told me was when he was a truck driver, in his younger days. He drove down Sutton Bank in Yorkshire, a notoriously steep hill that had a side sand track for truck drivers whose brakes fail. He had stopped at the bottom after deciding to put a tarp over the truck's tray because of a looming storm. He climbed onto the top of the truck and started to unfold the tarp. As he pulled it, walking backwards, he lost his footing and fell down onto the road. He landed on his arm, suffering great pain. A doctor told him he had a withered arm, meaning it would not recover and simply waste away to become a useless appendage. Don decided he'd treat himself, and was successful.

My aunt, living in Dublin, had a long standing case of allergy symptoms, but her doctor couldn't tell her what caused it. I recommended she saw Don who found that she was allergic to her gold jewellery. Her allergies disappeared when she stopped wearing anything made of gold.

I asked Don how his healing gift started. He said he came to realise he had a healing gift when visiting his mother during the war. Being confronted with almost certain death may have precipitated it, though he also told how his mother, when very pregnant with him, had gone to a local healer called Jack Rachford for treatment of a minor condition. After treating her, he told her that her boy child would be a world famous healer of sickness. This, in the days before scans revealed the gender.

At age 17 he lied about his age so he could join the airforce in WW2. Months later, at 18, he was a rear gunner in a Lancaster bomber flying over Germany. On one trip, their plane was caught in the focus of three searchlights and the ensuing flak was so intense the plane was being ripped apart. Sitting in the gun turret, alone from the rest of the crew, he feared the plane was going to crash. He closed his eyes and prayed. In Don's own words, *"It was exactly as though a door in my mind had been opened."* Then he heard a kind and gentle voice ring through his mind, saying, *"You are alright, my son, for I am with you."*

The plane did manage to limp back to England with much structural damage including large holes in the fuselage and wings. Taking time off after such a punishing event, Don went home to Yorkshire where he found his mother ill in bed. He went in to greet her and gave her a kiss on her cheek, putting a hand on her forehead as he did so. When he straightened up, his mother said, *"Oh Don, put your hand back, it feels so good."*

That became the moment of realisation that his touch was more than a mere touch. His mother told her friends and relatives and before long, Don found himself a reluctant healer - reluctant in that he wasn't immediately sure of himself being able to change anything by his touch.

There was always much humour around Don, as when a dentist, being treated in his Bradford terraced house sanctuary, suddenly grabbed Don's wrists and quickly pulled up his shirt sleeves, looking for the wires that must be producing the heat he felt during treatment. He was confused to find no wires.

Don's healing gift consumed his days for the rest of his life. He never advertised himself — all was by word of mouth. He was available 24/7 and treated tens of thousands of people. People from all walks of life came to him, often as a last resort, as was the case with myself. I remember once hearing how a group of housewives in America heard about Don and together, filled a plane and flew to Bradford, England, just to be treated by him.

Once, Don travelled to the Isle of Skye to visit me and my family. He brought his hang-glider, of course. I asked if I could fly it, not having my own. I took off over a steepish downward slope, forgetting to check and adjust the rigging. The resulting slightly painful flight caused great amusement as I skimmed the heather with my legs up and my bum down. At least, I think I hold the record for being the first person to hang-glide on the

Isle of Skye. The date was 1978. It was on that visit he talked about the pressure and responsibility he felt to heal. He said that he once stood in his garden on Greenbank Lane, in the dark, looking up at the sky, saying, *"Why me? Why me?"*

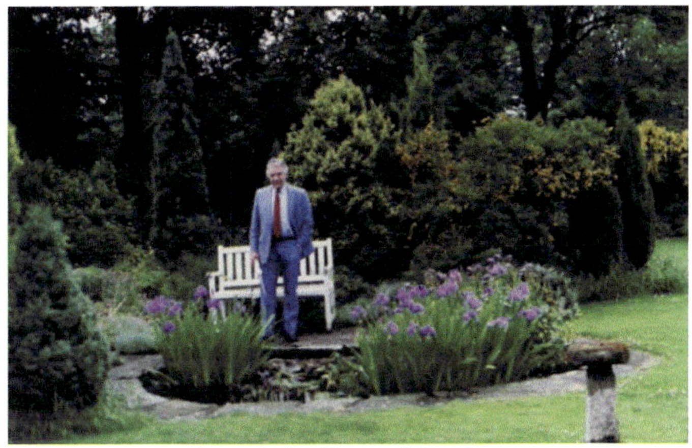

Don enjoying his peaceful garden.
Image by author P.A.Brown

To this day, I am thankful I met Don. I am indebted to him. My life would otherwise have worked out so very differently.

REFERENCES/LINKS

[1] Don's whisky habit eventually changed to drinking copious amounts of tea.

[2] *"A Healer's Pathway: The Man with the Power to Heal"* Ch3 p55 1992.

[3] Search: *"Dales Hang Gliding & Paragliding Club pub.Feb. 2007" (scroll to "Memories of Hang Gliding Early Days, Mike Shaw").*

Chapter Four

GORDON OF KHARTOUM

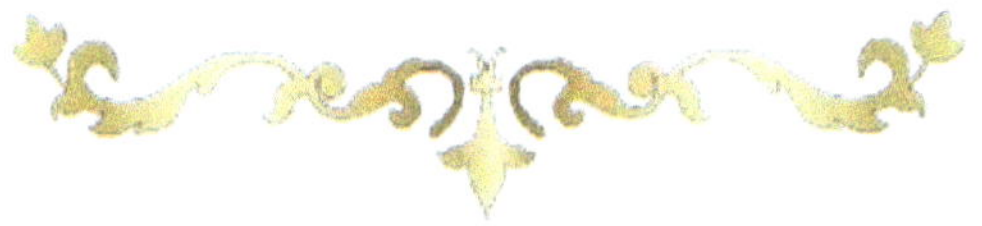

Indefatigable Reluctant Soldier

(1835-1885)

"If my life has a single point, it's this: I've learned to be unafraid of death but never to be unafraid of failure." Gen. Charles 'Chinese' Gordon.

Major-General Charles George Gordon was, by any yardstick, an extraordinary human being. As a child growing up in Yorkshire, my parents would regularly take me and my older brother to Harrogate, near York. We would visit two ageing aunts and spend the afternoon with them. The aunts always remembered my brother and I at Christmas with a little gift for each of us. After Christmas, my mother would always ask if we had remembered to write our thank-you letters to the Gordons in Harrogate. As a teen, I learned more about my aunts, Gwen and Violet. Violet Gordon was at one time a Senior Inspector of schools in the West Riding of Yorkshire and published a book in 1965 called, *"What Happens in School."* I still have my copy.

I remember hearing that the sisters travelled a lot. That appealed to me. Later, I heard that the sisters, in their 90's, had travelled to China for a holiday. I was impressed.

A few times my father talked about another Gordon relative. He said he was a very famous soldier. I was interested to find out more, but researching in the mid 1900's was not as easy as it is now. It was a case of visiting the library, talking to people or writing to people.

So when my parents succumbed to a persuasive Encyclopaedia Brittanica salesman, I became an avid reader of our very own precious set of 12 volumes about the world. I found references to Gordon of Khartoum and began to join the dots. That's when I first began feeling a connection, albeit tenuous, to a very popular and famous British soldier.

He is regarded as one of Britain's greatest military heroes but commanded Chinese, Egyptian and African troops, never British troops — an anomaly in British Military history.

So just how famous is he? Well, one way is to ask if there are any statues or memorials in his memory. In a word—lots!

Of statues, they include one in London (originally placed in Trafalgar Square, now on the embankment). Others are at: Brompton Barracks in Chatham; Gravesham in NW Kent; Woking, Surrey; Southampton, and memorials to him in Rochester Cathedral.

There is a most impressive tomb[1] in honour of him in St Paul's Cathedral, surely one of the grandest of all.

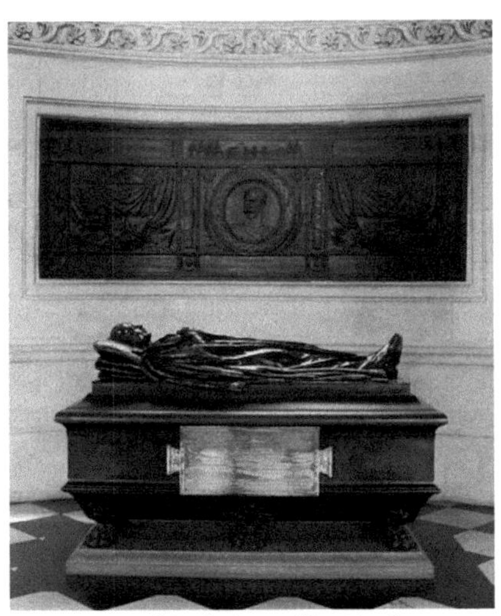

General Gordon's magnificent tomb at St Paul's Cathedral.
Sculptor Frederick William Pomeroy (1857-1924)

There are also statues in Aberdeen, Scotland and Melbourne, Australia. The statue with the most interesting and unlikely history is Gordon's Camel Statue. It was erected in 1902 at St Martin's Place, London. Then, in 1904 it was shipped to Khartoum, but temporarily sank in the Thames after a collision and also sank in the Nile on its final leg to Khartoum. In1958 when the Sudan had become independent, it was shipped back to England and in 1959 erected in its new and permanent home at Gordon's School. Formerly called The Gordon's Boy's School since 1943, it changed to Gordon's School in 1993 when it became co-educational. Prior to 1943, The Gordon Boys' School had been called The Gordon's Boy's Home, established in 1885, the same year that Gordon was killed in Khartoum. It was the National Memorial to General Gordon, and the idea is thought to have come from Queen Victoria herself. The reigning monarch of the UK has been a patron ever since.

While still a boy, Charle's spinster aunt Amy gave him a bible which was presented to the Queen after his death.

In more recent times, 2013, the school became an academy and rated outstanding by Ofsted (UK Office for Standards in Education) which monitors standards in schools by regular inspections.

Other schools and institutions in Gordon's memory include the Gordon Memorial College in Khartoum. Then, in Australia, in the city of Geelong, Victoria, is the Gordon Technical College. This was later renamed the Gordon Institute of Technology. Part of this Institute is known as the Gordon Institute of TAFE, the largest stand-alone TAFE in Victoria. The remainder of the institute was integrated with the Geelong State College, now known as Deakin University.

Other than all these statues, memorials, schools and institutions, there are other notable archival materials that record his qualities, military successes and awards. One is the little known fact that Gordon's death prompted the first dispatch of Australian troops overseas. Another is from Professor T.H.Huxley (1825-1895) — a leading English biologist and anthropologist who specialised in comparative anatomy. He became known as Darwin's Bulldog because of his defence of Darwin's theory of evolution. He wrote to a friend about Gordon, saying, quote: *"Of all the people I have ever met, he and Darwin were two in whom I found something bigger than the ordinary humanity, an unequalled simplicity and directness of purpose — a sublime unselfishness."*[2]

Another very surprising one, at least to me, is that after visiting Palestine in 1882-83, he suggested a different location for Golgotha, or Calvary, the site of Christ's crucifixion, to the traditional site a little northwards of the sepulchre. This site is known as 'The Garden Tomb' and has since been called by some, 'Gordon's Calvary' as it is regarded by many as a more logical location.

Nicknames given to Gordon reveal much of his illustrious military career. In chronological order, they are; Chinese

Gordon, Gordon Pasha and Gordon of Khartoum. However, before he earned these nick-names later in life, he was well know in his formative years at school for mischievous stunts and escapades. More of that later.

He was born in Woolwich January 28th, 1833 and interestingly, hated the roar of cannon which could often be heard from the arsenal nearby. He would put his fingers in his ears to cut out the noise. Over the years growing up, his father, together with the family, was stationed in Dublin, then Edinburgh and then Corfu. Charles, by then, was 7 years old. Here he learned to swim like a fish and overcame his reaction to gunfire and loud noises. Reaching the age of 10 in Corfu, he was brought home to England by his mother. He attended school at Taunton for the next 5 years. Academically Charles was slow but thorough. A letter he wrote at the age of 12 to a relative showed some perhaps surprising spelling errors. The Gordon family continued to grow in size. Eventually, there were 6 boys and 5 girls.

Here began that earlier mentioned and very noticeable characteristic of Charles Gordon— mischievous stunts and escapades which, as he grew older, turned into a reluctance to follow orders. To his credit, he was brave in never evading his punishments. In fact, on a few occasions after becoming a cadet at Woolwich, he came close to being dismissed from his career.

A memorable prank involved a plague of mice. He and his family's house in Woolwich was overrun with them. With his brother Henry, and sister Helen, they laid traps and caught a large number alive. One night, using baskets, the two boys slipped across the road in the darkness to the commandant's house which was opposite to theirs. They found an unlocked door and emptied the mice inside, then closed the door and quietly made their way back home, scarcely able to hold back their laughter.

A more extreme example of his pranks, in the sense that he would surely have been dismissed if caught, was more daring and possibly dangerous. As junior cadets, he and his brother and all the other junior cadets, were often teased and bullied by the senior cadets. Noticing an earth rampart had been built close by the room where the senior cadets attended lectures on certain evenings of the week, the boys hid behind the rampart with a pile of small stones they had collected.

The lecture was interrupted in a spectacular way. Suddenly, windows rattled as they were showered by small stones—some accounts say the windows shattered. These senior cadets reacted quickly and were in hot pursuit of whoever had vandalised the lecture room. Fortunately Charles and Henry were very familiar with every little detail of the grounds and managed to evade capture and certain dismissal.

At 19 Charles was given a commission as 2nd Lieutenant in the Engineers and stationed at Chatham for 2 years. In spite of some discovered pranks he had earned good conduct awards and was noted for his skills in fortifications and surveying. His father was apparently relieved that at last his son was going to be involved in real work and that his 3 years at Woolwich had proved worthwhile. His father described those 3 years as like sitting on a powder keg—a reference to Charles' many run-ins with authority.

During his second year as an engineer, the Crimean war broke out. He was ordered to Balaclava, arriving January 1st, 1885. His job was being in charge of materials for building wooden huts for the allied English, French and Turkish troops who were suffering very badly. Food was scarce and soldiers were freezing to death in the trenches. Shortly after this he was himself sent into the trenches close by Sebastopol. He and his comrades were under constant fire with hardly any time off duty.

As the war with the Russians continued, the assaults on Sebastopol intensified. The English Generals saw how their young officers coped and decided what particular duties they were adept at. The young Gordon was noticed for his boundless energy, courage, and an uncanny knack of correctly guessing what the Russians were doing, though not all of that was guesswork. He would crawl towards the enemy beyond the trenches, and observe what the Russians were up to. It is recorded Charles once did 34 consecutive 24 hour periods in the trenches which he described as 'a bit tedious'.

Eventually the Russians were pushed back and peace made. Charles was mentioned in despatches by the generals but not promoted, though received the Legion of Honour from the French.

After almost a full year in the Crimea he was ordered back home where he quickly earned his captaincy, working at Chatham. It was during his time in the Crimean war that Charles started to smoke. Smoking was unknown in Britain till the Crimean war. The Turks introduced the British troops to smoking. It became a thing that officers smoked cigars and lower ranks smoked cigarettes. Charles unusually smoked both cigars and Turkish cigarettes and became almost a chain smoker.

In 1860 the third China War started in order to enforce the Chinese ratification of the Treaty of Tientism which had resulted in the end of the 2nd Chinese War in 1859. The French and British organised a force that was intending to march on Peking. Charles, at the age of 27, volunteered and left in July 1860. By the time he arrived in Hong Kong, in September, he learned the Chinese Imperial Government was promising to sign the Treaty.

Arriving at the British camp near Tientsin in early October he was assigned command of a Royal Engineer company. The Chinese, meanwhile, had taken the diplomatic mediators prisoner, and so the war resumed. The British and French force prepared to break through the defences of Peking, but at the last moment, the Chinese surrendered, but not before the torture and executions of many of the prisoners. The surviving prisoners were released but the Allies decided to punish the

Emperor by ransacking, pillaging and torching the Summer Palace. The impressive, sumptuous, lavish and massive palace was thoroughly looted of removable items before it was set on fire.

Charles wrote a description of the magnificence of what he saw. He himself purchased, for next to nothing, a most impressive throne which he presented to Brompton Barracks in Chatham and is apparently still there to this day. However, Charles wrote about the demoralising effect of all this and when he later achieved independent command, he never permitted looting.

The Allies stationed 3,000 soldiers at Tientsin until the Chinese paid all of the agreed surety. Charles was made Commander Royal Engineers of the British brigade. Charles liked his appointment and wrote to friends in England that he liked this place very much and didn't want to return to England, though asked those he told, to please not mention it to his parents.

One thing that Charles regretted deeply was the poverty. He managed a relief fund, possibly of his own making. However the Mandarins refused to help organise a controlled distribution for the poorest people, so Charles organised a day for this and around 3,000 arrived. In the crush 7 women and a boy were killed. I wonder if the Mandarins battered an eyelid?

The conflicts in China around this time are so complex and interwoven, it is a subject in its own right. Briefly, for 30 years before these times, the lower classes and peasants were greatly disgruntled with the government. They had suffered floods, famine and high taxation—the seeds of rebellion. A 36 years old farmer's son, named Hung Hsui-chuan, started a religious movement, based on a confused understanding of Christianity. He declared himself the Heavenly King. It attracted immediate support, fuelled by their dislike of how in the 17th Century the Ming dynasty had been overthrown by foreigners who established the Ching dynasty. It rapidly turned into a nationalistic movement.

This insurrection became known as the Taeping rebellion. The government was very slow to react which allowed the movement to grow. The Taiping armies moved northwards, taking city after city.

Hung Hsui-chuan taught his followers the Ten Commandments and that he was the younger brother of Jesus. Western missionaries in China, forbidden by the government to evangelise beyond the Treaty Ports, heard about this Heavenly King and thought that an indigenous Christian movement had begun. This even created a lobby group in England with some believing that China was about to become a Christian country. An amusing thought in retrospect.

The rebellion set its sights on taking Shanghai. The western merchants and Chinese bankers were fearful of this and so put forward funds to raise a Chinese army led by foreign officers. The Chinese, in hope, named this new force The Ever

Victorious Army. A 29 years old American called Ward took control of this new army but most of the European officers he chose to lead the Chinese soldiers were not military-trained at all. They were volunteers from out-of-work seamen, bored office workers and a few army deserters. Many of them drank far too much, too. To their credit, they won a few small battles, but it hardly seemed they were going to provide the solution.

Then a British officer, Charles Stavely, left Tientsin and arrived in Shanghai with orders to command a small British force defending the International Settlement—an obvious attempt to protect and maintain trade with China. His orders were to drive the Taiping rebels well away from the city. He chose Charles Gordon to be his Commander Royal Engineers.

Charles arrived in Shanghai in May 1862 and immediately started work. Stavely said of Gordon, years later, that he was invaluable in his tasks though caused much anxiety by his daring ways of getting close to the enemy to obtain information.

When news of Ward's death in battle reached the British Consul in Shanghai, it was suggested that a British officer should replace Ward. Here was yet another long list of interwoven complications in this Chinese War story. To step over all the fine details, Charles Gordon was eventually established as the new leader of the Ever Victorious Army, a post that was way above his rank. At the same time, he remained a British officer, on loan to the Chinese Government.

Charles proved himself more than capable and it was noted how he exhibited extraordinary powers to lead indigenous troops. That, with his already well-noted abilities in reconnaissance and exceptional daring proved disastrous to the Taipings, who gave up their siege in that area rather than face Charles again.

Charles gave up his salary from the Chinese government to help pay his soldiers who were often not paid on time. While this could never solve the problem the gesture was not lost on the soldiers. He prohibited looting and killing of prisoners, on pain of death. However, this was not the end of the Taipan rebellion. Far from it. For Charles this was the beginning of his work in China.

After many more serious battles, twists and massacres beyond his control, Charles finally left China on 25th November, 1964, 3 months after the Ever Victorious Army was fully disbanded. He left as poor as he entered, though it's estimated he saved around 100,000 lives. The rebellion took 20-30 million lives (some estimates say up to 100 million). For comparison, WW2 lives lost was 17 million.

The Chinese government gave him the highest military honour, normally reserved only for Chinese mandarins, and not many of these awards have been given. One source mentioned 14, another, 21. He remains the only non-Chinese person to be honoured with the Hang Ma-Kwa (Yellow Jacket).[3] The legend of Chinese Gordon was thus endorsed by the Chinese with this most significant gesture.

It occurs to me that if ever a film director was to try to make a film about Chinese Gordon, of his time in China, he would have an almost impossible task of writing a coherent plot that audiences would be able to follow. I have read three books on the subject and I am still trying to put all the pieces into a coherent whole. The word 'complex' isn't enough! Charles seemed to always be in more than one place at a time, without resting.

The film 'Khartoum' of 1966, very dated by now, gives quite an accurate account of his time in Khartoum, except for one detail—General Gordon didn't meet the Madhi face to face, though they did communicate.

Some unusual actions of Charles at home and abroad demonstrate his most generous spirit:

- When an American officer had been caught red-handed communicating with the enemy in China, Gordon's punishment was for the officer to lead the next foray forward. The American caught a bullet in his mouth and fell ... into Charles' arms, close by.

- When a young Chinese soldier on the front line was shaking with fear as he tried to aim his rifle, Charles knelt at his side and put the rifle barrel on his own shoulder to steady the soldier's aim.

- Whenever Charles went into action, he never hesitated

to be on the frontline, unarmed, smoking a cigar with a cane in his other hand. He did this in the Crimea, China and Africa. He seemed to lead a charmed life and some soldiers believed his cane magically stopped him being hit by bullets.

- In the battle to retake the city of Quinsan, Charles had an infant clinging to his leg. Gordon looked after him as well as he could during the fighting, then had the child sent to Shanghai, arranging for a foster parent and paying for his education. Charles called him Quincey. Later on Quincey became Shanghai's Nanking railway chief of police. He started a family from which, 130 years later a woman became an academic in America.

- When in England Charles spent most of his time in Gravesend where there was much poverty. He took provisions to starving families, visiting sick people and doing a few chores for them. He spent time with the street urchins allowing them to make free with his garden and house where he taught them geography and was able to help them find work. He had a large wall map of the world in a room for the children to plot where some of the older ones in merchant shipping had sailed, since finding work.

- With his housekeeper's help, he used 2 of his rooms as

classrooms and basic resource rooms for boys living on the streets. He also rented a small house for working boys to be taught for free.

- Every year Charles gave away around 90% of his income to charity.

- He found an East End boy with symptoms of tuberculosis and sent him to Margate for open-air treatment at his own expense.

- He let his neighbours use his garden to grow fruit and vegetables.

Charles' time in Africa was equally, if not more complicated, than his time in China. Everywhere, he found fever, laziness, discontent and frequent rebellion.

From the khedive in Cairo, he accepted the position of Governor of the Equatorial Provinces, accepting a salary of L2,000 a year, instead of the L10,000 offered. After two years of very trying times and conditions, Charles had gained trust from most of the natives. He made sure his men took nothing from them without payment. He even found time, between capturing convoys of slaves, to visit an old, dying native woman, providing her with food and company. Previous to this the Egyptian Governor had made the natives work without pay. The Egyptian officials, more often than not, sided with the slave-traders, taking bribes, and, he found, plotting against him.

At the end of these two years he resigned his position and returned to England. The khedive, however, had other plans. As soon as he arrived in England, frequent telegrams implored him to go back and continue his work. After only 6 weeks, he did return and on meeting the khedive, he said he would not continue unless he was granted full authority and power over the Sudan and the other provinces. The khedive agree to all Charles' demands and Ismail Pasha, the governor-general of the Sudan, was recalled. Charles took his place as ruler over all the equatorial provinces—Darfour, all the Sudan and the Red Sea coast. He would answer to no-one but the khedive, who was, in turn, subordinate to the sultan of Turkey. The khedive offered Charles a salary of L12,000 a year, but he accepted only L6,000 and later cut this down to only L3,000.

One account of Charles' many dangerous negotiations in Africa illustrates as well as any his totally unselfish commitment to his often impossibly difficult work. Remembering that Charles was instrumental in the creation of the Anglo-Egyption Convention for the suppression of the slave trade, signed in 1877, Charles was still doing everything in his power to break the slave trade years later. In 1879 he reluctantly agreed to go to Abyssinia where a peace treaty was to be signed by King John.

For some perspective of the kind of person King John was, unfortunately makes for unpleasant reading. He variously cut off noses, ears or hands, and put out eyes of anyone who displeased him. Charles described him "... *as a man of most disagreeable expression, never smiles or looks you in face, suspicious of everyone, without friends, hating and hated of all."*

To reach King John, Charles rode a mule for 38 days, through what he described as interminable mountains and sheep tracks that the locals called roads, finally arriving at the capital, Debra Tabor near Mandala.

After only 3 minutes, Charles was dismissed by King John. The next day Charles spent a little longer talking to him. King John demanded that if he was to sign a peace treaty, he must be given ownership of 5 districts, an indemnity, and a Coptic Archbishop from Alexandria to come and crown him.

Charles then asked King John to write his demands in a letter and allow 6 months for a reply. At some risk, one can assume, Charles said he didn't think Egypt was likely to agree to the terms! The king became angry and asked Charles if he realised he could be killed on the spot. King John was staggered by Charles' reply. *"I am perfectly well aware of it, your Majesty. Do so at once if it is your royal pleasure. I am ready."*

The king refused to release 8 Egyptian prisoners and tried to bribe Charles to desert the khedive. After all this the king did write the letter, though it proved to be insulting.

Charles' journey back was deliberately made difficult by allowing Charles to spend days on his mule until reaching a hill from where he could see his own territory, but then apprehended by one of the king's governors, under orders to make Charles return and go back by another, longer route out of Abyssinia. He had to endure being bullied and hindered, travel through snow and frost, give up his tent as a bribe, get arrested and robbed at the frontier, then finally released, arriving sick and exhausted at Massawa. The return trip had taken 89 days, 79 on his mule and expensive presents to the king and bribes getting out of the country.

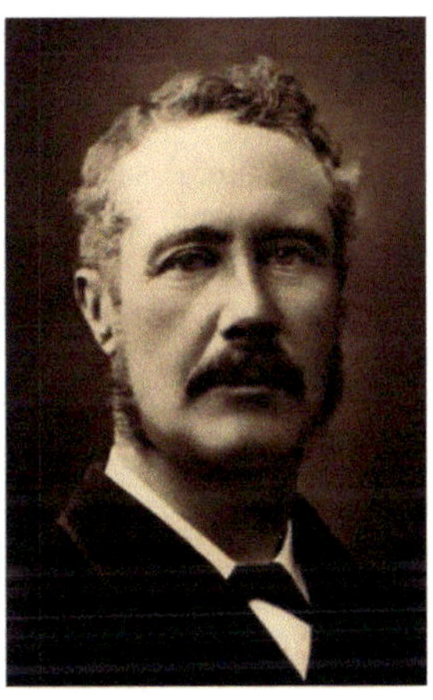

General Gordon at age 44
Attribution: Geruzet Frères (active c.1870-1889) Date:1887

This short account of Major General Gordon covers only a fraction of his life's endeavours, trials and tribulations. The story of his end in Khartoum at the hands of the Madhi's army is well known by most, who have, no doubt, seen the picture by the artist G. W. Joy, of Charles' death as he descended the steps of the palace. A spear pierces his chest and he falls dead.

His manner of death, however, is disputed. There are a few accounts. One says he was shot with a bullet in an open space near the palace, walking with a group of people towards the

Austrian consul's house. Perhaps the most convincing account is that told by an Englishman 43 years later, talking to an elderly man in a group of people on the East bank of the Blue Nile. This man said he saw Gordon die. He described Gordon standing unarmed at the top of the palace steps. He said Charles tore open his tunic and said, *"Strike! Strike hard!"* and somebody threw a spear.

What is certain is his head was paraded through the streets of Khartoum on the end of a pike. A sad end to a true champion of the downtrodden, slaves and persecuted people in China and Africa. I will always be in awe of this man. What he achieved in his life of 51 years seems vastly underrated and now forgotten by most.

REFERENCES/LINKS

[1] Search: Gordon's tomb, St Paul's

[2] Brief Biographies No.13 p4 Hanson. Lutterworth Press 1950 (out of print)

[3] John Pollock's book: *"Gordon of Khartoum. An Extraordinary Soldier"* p130

The British Museum carries a huge store of Charles' writings.

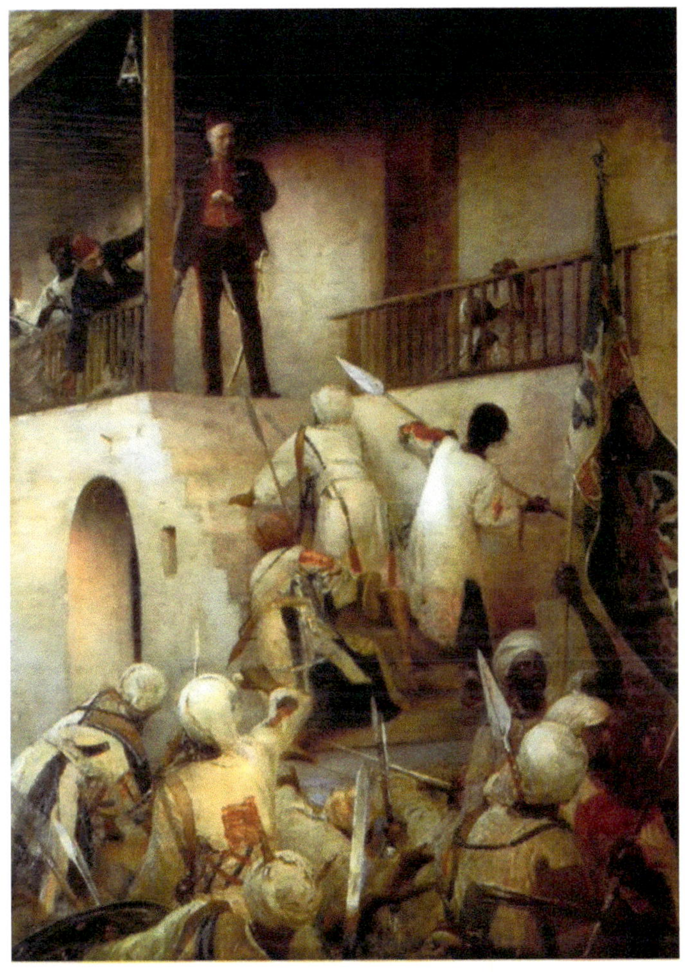

General Gordon's Last Stand

By George W. Joy (1844-1925) Public Domain

Chapter Five

SIR GEOFROY TORY

Dowser Extraordinaire

(1912-2012)

Presenter: *Mick, how do you feel about dowsing?*

Mick Aston: *Sceptical*

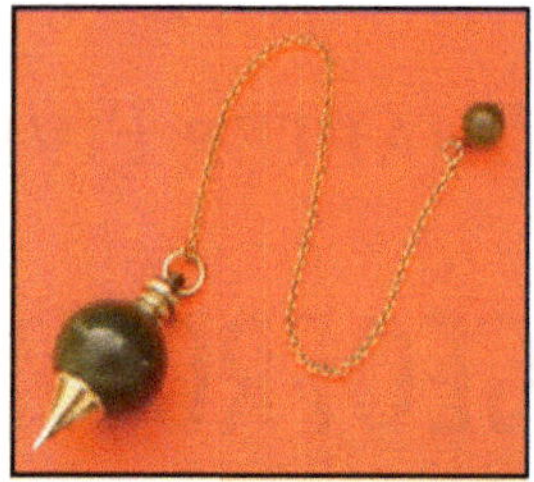

When I first met Geofroy I knew nothing about him except he was the father of a friend and that he dowsed. At the time, I was becoming aware that dowsing was a wider subject than just searching for water. I had tried using a pendulum with a few surprising results and so any further experiences were welcome.

In the 70's I was living on the Isle of Skye and had reason to believe that a small conical hill near my place of work might be a tumulus rather than natural.

Geofroy's daughter visited my family and I, and the conical hill was talked about. We tried a bit of dowsing, with twigs. She suggested drawing a sketch of the hill and sending it to her father to dowse.

This I did and within 3 weeks I received a letter and my sketch map with added information. In the letter he said the hill had a few points of interest, which he had marked on the map. It showed a confluence of three underground streams of water under the high point of the hill. He wrote that he was sure the hill was a tumulus and marked on the map the entry and position of the monolithic stones of the grave. It was on the north-eastern slope of the hill and not directly under the high point of the hill.

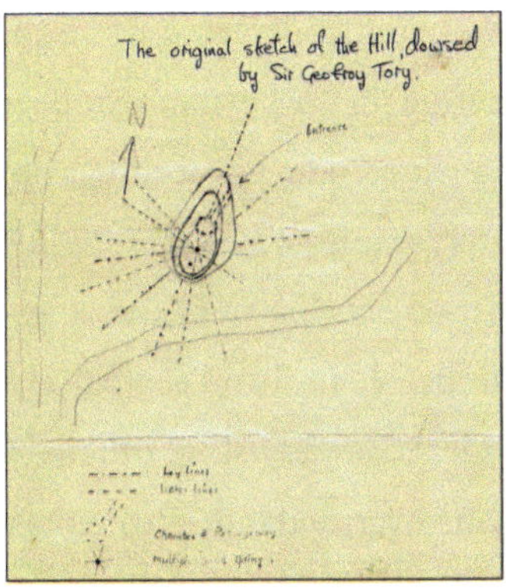

The original sketch of the Fairy Hill on Isle of Skye, Scotland, dowsed by Sir Geofroy Tory.
Image copyright author. Original sketch by author.

Years later, a friend of mine on Rapa Nui (Easter Island) asked me if I had any ideas on how to find water on an area of land his family owned. I drew a sketch from his documents and sent it to Geofroy. He dowsed the map and found only one underground stream. The island is composed of much limestone, so surface water is a rarity, making wells a necessity.

But what does science have to say about dowsing? Well, not much. It seems like it doesn't want to consider it. Some scientists accept it as something that can't currently be explained by traditional ways of scientific investigation. Others, however, the majority, scoff at the suggestion there is anything in it at all.

When pressed, they offer explanations like dowsers associate different kinds of environments and geology with the likelihood of there being underground streams there. Of course these scientists deride the suggestion that people can dowse for things other than water. The list of things dowsed, besides the main one of water, seems endless; buried metal objects, ores, oil, gravesites, lost objects like keys and rings, lost pets, and in modern times, archaeological and geological work.

Many countries use dowsing officially. That is, they employ workers in government departments who regularly use dowsing as part of their job. An example is a former government worker between1925 and 1930 called Major Pogson who was the Official Water Diviner for the Government of India. His advice was sought on everything to do with underground water. A more recent example is in Carmel Valley, California, where the telephone company has a dowser on call.

Nigel Percy of the Canadian Society of Dowsers wrote a sound, well founded article[1] called, " Dowsing and Science — An Inevitable Partnership?" In it he says that when the critiques of science are examined, it is clear that science itself is based on a subjective interaction of the observer with the world.

"Subjective" is the key word there. So just because science can't justify dowsing in scientific terminology doesn't preclude its existence. One look at recent findings in astronomy confirms science is in a continuous learning curve of surprises.

There is even disagreement about when dowsing began. Evidence of dowsing in ancient times is scarce but not absent. The World Heritage Tassel Cave pictographs in southern Algeria, numbering over 15,000, are dated at around 10,000 BC and one picture[2&4] clearly shows a person holding a forked rod in front of him in a typical dowsing stance. The ancient Egyptians and Chinese are recorded as practising dowsing. Celtic druids and people in the Middle Ages used it.

Homer's Odyssey talks about Circe using a rhabdos, Greek for rod. Cicero, a Roman elder statesman, called this kind of rod a virgula divina, which translates to divine rod.

There was extensive use of dowsing in 15th Century Germany to find metals. In 17th century France it was used for identifying law breakers and heretics though one wonders how successful that was!

Over such a very long history, dowsing, unsurprisingly, has had various names, such as, divining, water-witching, doodle-bugging (used for petroleum searches), water- smelling, peach-twig toting, well-prophesying, rhabdomancy and radiesthesie. This last one was coined in France in the 1930's when using a pendulum instead of a rod. The word dowsing itself came into common use in England in the 17th century.

Martin Luther no doubt witnessed the art because he condemned it as witchcraft. The Catholic Church totally banned it, probably because they couldn't understand it and like Luther, imputed something evil must be involved. Lloyd Youngblood of the American Society of Dowsers, wrote that on research trips to Egypt and the Middle East he has photographed 4000 year old temple walls showing pharaohs holding what appear to be divining rods. He goes on to say that in the Cairo museum there are ceramic pendulums, removed from ancient tombs.

Conventional scientific investigation methods have no explanation as to how some dowsers' sensitivity enables them to predict the depth and quantity of water available in a particular spot. And this is a regular feature of water divining.

Find a scientist willing to discuss dowsing and the part of dowsing that will irritate them the most, because they can't do this with their scientific equipment, is to explain how dowsers can locate the exact spot to drill, the exact depth to drill to, describe the quality of the water and even the volume of output per hour. This is regularly observed and recorded.

Dan Schwartz, a journalist, wrote an excellent article about Leroy Bull[3], regarded as the pre-eminent dowser of the USA. Leroy's abilities equate well with Sir Geofroy's dowsing skills and stories. In the article another dowser, Herbert, is mentioned as using an unusual pendulum called an aura meter, "*... an elaborate pendulum that resembles a chrome heron with a spring-loaded neck that bobbles in different directions to answer questions. It's the Cadillac of dowsing tools, he says.*"

Personally, I am not interested in esoteric and argumentative discussions about whether dowsing is scientifically verifiable. Having personal experiences that defy scientific rationalisation is proof enough. Besides, only the ignorant would casually knock dowsing as obscure nonsense. Would they reconsider if they knew that Einstein was a dowser? He acknowledged science had no explanation for it but that one day it would. Other scientists who dowsed, and most people are likely unaware they did, are Thomas Edison, Sir Isaac Newton and Leonardo da Vinci.[4]

Geofroy delighted me with the return of my sketch of the hill near my place of work on Skye. I couldn't prove by digging whether three streams did converge there and if a tumulus-style grave was inside. I sought permission and was encouraged by Lord MacDonald, the Laird, but was prevented by local official restrictions. These, I think, seemed more an aversion to disturbing this hill, named Cnoc Sithean (Fairy Hill in English), likely because of unspoken superstition about it needing to remain undisturbed. The Gaelic name 'sithean' is used to name small conical hills and in Celtic mythology they were believed to have hollow interiors where lived fairies or 'wee folk' as they are known, and where unbaptised children were taken.

On another occasion, I had a story recounted to me of a social evening at Geofroy's place in Ireland. It was a balmy evening and after dinner everyone had gone outside to enjoy the fresh air. Close by was a paddock with grass about 30cm high.

Someone asked a woman if they could borrow her wedding ring for a while, and was assured it would be returned. With some hesitation the ring was handed over and imagine her shock to see it immediately tossed into the grassy paddock. Then Geofroy, who was chatting with another group of people, was called over to find a lost wedding ring 'dropped' in the paddock. He apparently was a little annoyed to have to parade his dowsing skills in front of a crowd, but saw the need to recover the ring. It took him a little more than 5 minutes to find it.

On another occasion, years later, I was visiting Ireland and one evening was sitting at the dining table at Wendy's house. Her boyfriend was sitting to my left and Wendy was standing near the ovens while her father, Geofroy, was sitting opposite me. He was hunched over something he was holding just under the table top.

Wendy said, *"Oh dad! What are you doing?"*

"Oh nothing, just dowsing Philip."

This was my first personal experience of health diagnosis by dowsing. He rated me as quite healthy and having nothing untoward lurking or emerging.

Once, years later again, while travelling in South America, Daniel Bruin W. (Chapter 7) asked me if I knew anything about being allergic to wheat. He said an Argentinian friend's wife had some allergy that was causing quite severe reactions and they were beginning to suspect it may be caused by the bread she ate. I suggested sending a hair sample to Geofroy to let him dowse it. This was done and several weeks later I was able to write to those people and tell them that Geofroy strongly suspected gluten intolerance. So they stopped eating wheat, rye and barley products and her allergy symptoms stopped. This was well before gluten intolerance became a common subject.

I saved Geofroy's crowning glory of his amazing dowsing abilities till last. He was a long serving and distinguished diplomat who had a breadth of interests and skills, namely a painter of portraits, a Fellow of the Royal Astronomical Society, beekeeper, wine maker and grafter of fruit seedlings. In his retirement he became fluent in Russian, Latin and Spanish. He assisted the gardaí, the Irish police in searches for bodies and diagnosed through dowsing over 400 people's allergies.

His most astonishing dowsing event, however, at least in my opinion, was something that happened when he was a diplomat. He had a friend working in the CIA with whom he would chat to on the phone from the UK. At this particular time, it was the Cold War, which lasted decades. Nuclear submarines were being built in increasing numbers from the late 1950's. At a time when Russia had only two nuclear submarines, the western countries naturally wanted to know where those submarines were at all times, if possible.

In a conversation by phone with his friend in the CIA one evening, Geofroy was asked if the British Government knew of the whereabouts of the Russian subs. Geofroy replied in the negative, but added that he could find out. His friend laughed, even scoffed, when Geofroy told him to expect a call within the next 24 hours. Geofroy took a world map and began dowsing for the 2 Russian subs. When he called his friend again he told him where the subs were and the incredulous voice of his friend asked him if he was being serious.

The upshot of this created quite a stir in the Pentagon as Geofroy's stated location of the subs later proved correct. The label I honour Sir Geofroy[5] with—Dowser Extraordinaire, is fully deserved.

REFERENCES/LINKS

[1] Search: *Dowsing and Science – an inevitable partnership?*

[2 & 4] Search: *Dowsing History-vibrational health*

[3] Search: *Dan Schwartz The Inexplicable World of Dowsing*

[5] *Search: Sir Geofroy Tory/wiki*

CHAPTER SIX

JOHN RODLEY

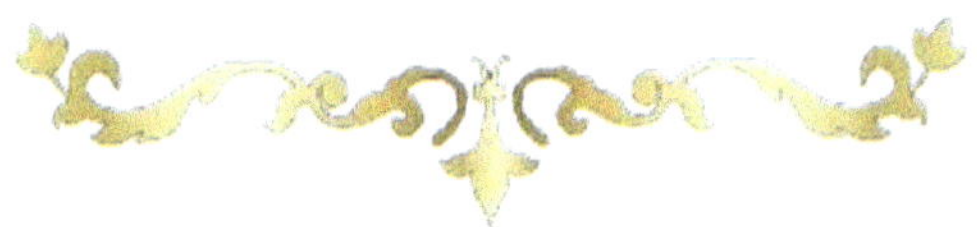

PAINTER, SCULPTOR, SOCIALITE

(circa 1940-1994)

" He who cares not what others think of him is truly a free person." Samuel Zulu.

I need to clear up at the outset my choice of the word 'socialite'. It's often used by the media to imply a slightly derogative nature. There was nothing derogatory about John. He was adept at socialising in any level of society without any pretence of airs and graces nor any attempt to look well dressed. What you saw was what you got.

I first met John in 1967, though can't remember the exact circumstances of our meeting. I had moved to Lincolnshire to take up work in Grimsby. I found a tiny village called Riby, a few miles from Grimsby, where I rented an interesting old house full of Maori objects and paintings.

John was an artist and sculptor living in a rather run down old mansion in Grimsby which he shared with his mother and sister. I never did learn anything else about his immediate family. I remain curious about what his father was like. The mansion had a separate building—an old coach house and stables from the days before vehicles. John told me that the stables had been where Marmite, the food spread, had been invented. A great and continuing commercial success!

At the time John showed me around, the converted stables had a tenant, an old woman he described as quite mad, who loved the weeds growing everywhere and could often be seen collecting them.

I have changed my view about her and no longer regard her as a mad old woman. Why? Because I grow my own weeds —

dandelions, nettles, and chickweed because of their incredible nutritional and therapeutic value.

John's appearance was always totally casual, in fact, not even what is known as 'smart casual'. I never saw him in a suit. I don't think he even owned one. John's life routine at that time was spending half the year at home, or at least in the UK somewhere, and the other half travelling abroad in his old diesel Trojan personnel carrier.[1] He'd been using this old vehicle for some years. He had made no attempt to sharpen its looks. I doubted it would ever be stolen!

Trojan's first vehicle dates from 1910. The model John had, dated from 1953, when Trojan became the first vehicle manufacturer to use a diesel engine in a 1 tonne van.

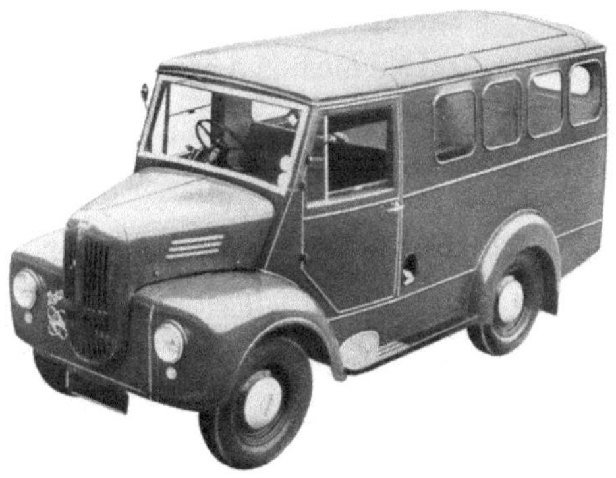

Trojan Diesel
Image courtesy David Hambleton, Trojan Museum Trust

It had not been an easy task, apparently, to persuade Perkins to let them use a 3 litre, 3 cylinder engine. It was, basically, a Perkins 6 cylinder engine, cut in half! John told me its advantages. It was ultra-reliable and easily adaptable to a camper-van, though he hated the word 'camper'. He described one trip to Spain as travelling into the countryside looking for a small village he liked the look of.

His routine at that point was to ask permission to park his vehicle for a few days and in return offered to paint murals on the exterior of the cottage walls. These were usually large, country scenes. He said he enjoyed the friendly evenings, sitting outside around a fire, playing his guitar and swapping stories with the villagers.

I was persuaded by John to look for an old Trojan Diesel van as he saw it would suit me fine. I eventually found my Trojan in the city of Bradford, Yorkshire, England. It was in a scrap yard, sitting on top of a pile of old vehicles around 5 metres high. The scrap yard owner told me it had been there for a couple of years. That meant it had weathered through two wet and snowy winters. Without checking anything out, I had already decided I wanted it while talking to the scrap yard over the phone. Scarcity was the main reason for my quick decision!

On the day I went to collect it, I took a new vehicle battery. A crane proceeded to lift the vehicle down. Someone reached into the cab and released the handbrake. The crane then dragged the vehicle across the ground to get the wheels moving freely as two were seized up. One was very stubborn but eventually was freed. I put in the new battery. The workers watched, bemused by my expectation of driving the vehicle out of the scrapyard.

I had paid the owner the agreed price of £25 then climbed into the driver's seat and switched on the ignition. Amazingly, the engine fired and started on the third try. The workers, looking surprised, grinned back at me. They happily checked my tyres and I drove it all the way home, though with some trepidation, as the brakes were not working too well and it wasn't yet registered.

This particular model had been converted for use as an ice cream van and so had standing-up room behind the front seats. And so began a 9 year affair with a vehicle already 19 years old. I converted the inside into a sort of camper-van with a cooker and bench seats that folded into beds. It proved to be a useful holiday vehicle for my young family though not a very convenient one for daily use. It attracted much attention.

John had a lot of social connections, many of which could be described as in high places. He once described to me a typical routine when he came back to the UK after being abroad for months, usually in Spain or France. He'd call up an acquaintance and invite himself over. One such visit, lasting a few days, involved going to a mansion of, and I'm being deliberately vague here, a landed gentleman as they are sometimes called. John rolled up in his old, hand-painted Trojan vehicle, and stayed there for a few days. He told me what his host said on the first morning, as he descended the stairs and entered the breakfast room. He lowered his newspaper and jovially shouted, *"Morning John. How was she?"*

He was referring to the fact that his wife and John had slept together. I hope that doesn't make me sound naive, as we all know this goes on at all levels of society, but to hear it unexpectedly at first hand surprised me.

Over the following year in Grimsby, John was occasionally in the local news for exhibitions that included his sculptures and paintings. Then one day he informed me he was going to Monte Carlo for a while. It was 1966 and a friend, the London based originator of the popular Fanny's Discotheque had asked John to model a building he'd just rented or purchased in Monte Carlo along the lines of his London discotheque. He wanted John to hire builder's labourers, supervise the renovations and to feel free to add his own ideas. The building was a stone's throw away from the famous casino, on the same road.

Not to be confused with the huge Jimmey'z Discotheque of Monte Carlo in later years, this was a small cafe-disco type of business. I admit to being confused about the name 'Fanny's' because I distinctly remember John calling the London one that, and the owner wanted his second disco place in Monaco to also be called Fanny's. An online search talks about a famous Fanny's at Newcastle, and not London. Confusing.

Serendipitously, as it turned out, I too was arranging to travel abroad—a new job in Kayseri, central Turkey. So John said to call in at Monte Carlo where he would be and, he worked out, maybe the discotheque would be up and running. So John left Grimsby while I bought a 2nd hand British Army Champ jeep[2] for the anticipated rough country in Central Turkey and made preparations to drive there from England. My then wife and I arrived in Monte Carlo a few days before the new disco was due to open.

That jeep, by the way, was, is, truly amazing. It is super strong and sturdy, has a Rolls Royce engine, fully water-proofed to allow the jeep to be driven in 6 feet of water when the breather tube is elevated, and can use any kind of petrol from the highest to lowest octane values without any difference in engine performance. I even successfully tested its ability to run on paraffin. This I did in Wales, on my return to UK from Turkey. The engine sounded and performed like it was using petrol. That was only a test and not to evade petrol tax! It also has a crawler gear that makes other vehicles with a low gear seem like they're in 1st and 2nd gear. It can also reverse faster than any car or jeep I've heard about. How? Because you can change gear going backwards! Army personnel in parade grounds would, if no-one higher up was watching, have backward driving races.

I recall hearing of a young guy who bought one and stripped off the army green paint job to customise it. Unfortunately, he lived in a terraced street of houses in England, without garages. He had to leave his jeep parked in the street for 3-4 months, stripped to the metal, because his job had called him away. The wet British weather tried its best to rust it out, without success! When the guy came back, expecting the worst, he found it just as he had left it, gleaming. Apparently, these jeeps were dipped in liquid cadmium before being painted British Army Green.

The building John helped establish and supervise its refurbishment as a disco, had some unusual elements for its time in the 1960's. Every surface save the table tops was matt black. This included the floors, walls and ceilings.

We had arrived in Monte Carlo just a few days prior to the scheduled opening night and had already been given a quick tour of the place by John. On opening night we drove there and were amazed to be able to park right outside.

John ushered us in and straightaway introduced a couple whose first names escape me now, but were the Spicers of Fine Paper fame. We sat together at a table and had drinks. I remember she had the longest fingernails I had ever seen, painted a bright green. They invited us to visit them the next day at their apartment overlooking the famous harbour, full of million dollar yachts.

The next day the three of us were entertained by the Spicers. He was keen to show John and me his collection of model train engines, each in their own glass case. They were quite large, about a metre in length. Later the couple resumed a discussion they had started before we arrived. It was about which type of new yacht they would soon be buying. His ideas were different to hers. They even started raising their voices about the difference in cost—around $15,000, which at that time was a lot of money. She pointed through the window to a yacht in the harbour, saying she wanted one like that.

Somewhere there in the harbour lay their current luxury yacht. I reflected later the wondrous, vastly different amounts of money argued over between couple's available finances. Mine would have been far less than a thousand.

A couple of days after meeting the Spicers, we were sitting outside Fanney's, now becoming popular, when the son of one of the biggest UK building companies happened by. John and he knew each other, so he joined us. John explained later that the young guy's father had insisted, for tax avoidance reason, that he live abroad for a few years. Monaco was his first pick—unsurprising with his level of wealth. Anyway, he parked his Porsche next to my British Army Champ jeep[2].

He asked John,"Who owns the jeep?

John nodded at me. The young guy, name withheld, asked me a few things about it and then popped the question, "Can I have a drive?"

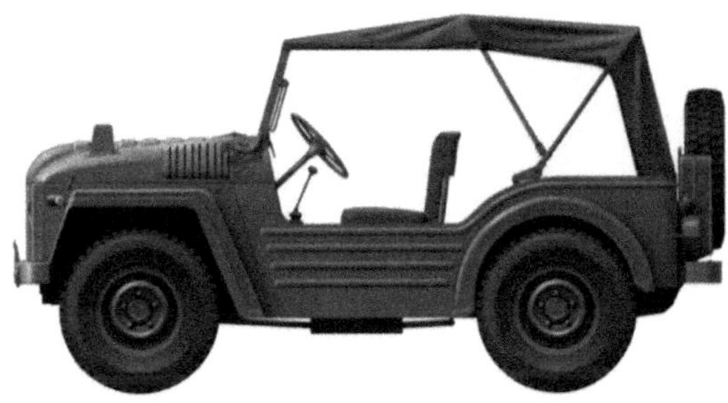

British Army Champ Jeep
Image courtesy of Ardhya Anargha, The Online Tank Museum

I remember looking at John while insurance and possible damage crossed my mind. With the hood and side-screens off, and the windscreen folded flat on the bonnet, he got his drive. Off he went. After about a quarter of an hour, he returned with a serious look on his face. He looked at John and said, *"Bloody hell, I got more attention driving that jeep than my Porsche."*

Over the coming weeks, the discotheque became even more popular. However, its success may have had as much to do with John himself than the disco. While in Monaco, he became publicly known for his appearances in a French television panel game. He was known as Jean la Barbe (John the Beard). His bushy beard and large stature did somehow give meaning to his nickname.

It was undoubtedly his popularity in the TV show that resulted in him being invited to the palace by Prince Rainier and Princess Grace. (I did describe him as a socialite, right!)

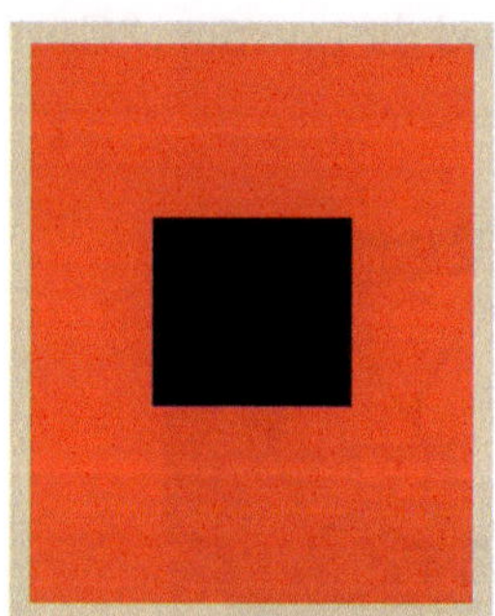

Computer image of John's quickly painted 'masterpiece' (in oils). Does it still hang in the palace?
Image by author

It must have been a successful evening because John told me he was invited back a second time! Besides his involvement in the new disco, his artwork was an obvious subject of conversation at the palace, which resulted in John painting an abstract for them which was hung somewhere in the palace. John laughed out loud when I asked him what the picture consisted of. He said he painted it in a single evening, while rather drunk. It was a large black square on a bright red background. In later years John gave me a copy. It came with me to Australia in 1981. One of many reminders of him.

While working in Monte Carlo, John was staying at a friend's place in Coaraze[3], a small medieval village in the Nice Hinterland of France, perched on a hill top with a population of under 900. John arranged for us to stay with him there, until we resumed our travel to Turkey. Years later I read Coaraze is a member of the Les Plus Beaux Villages de France (the association of the most beautiful villages of France). That came as no surprise at all, as it is architecturally a very attractive and unusual village, among magnificent scenery.

His friend, Bernard, was a frustrated painter turned successful sculptor, following John's suggestion to change tack a few years prior. Bernard and his family were memorable for many reasons. They lived with their two young children in a beautiful old house with a large, high walled courtyard which to them was their dining room with a spectacular view, many miles down into a large, forested valley.

At least once a week. Bernard would scan a particular site down in the valley with binoculars. John recounted a trip with Bernard to that site, a municipal dump. They went to recover a crate of large cheeses Bernard had watched being dumped. He knew that well inside the cheeses it would be perfectly useable. On bringing it back to the house, he cut off thick swathes of the outer layer of mouldy cheese to reveal the next month or two's supply of cheese for their family of four.

Bernard later achieved fame with a controversial display in London. I think, but not certain, it was the Museum of Contemporary Art. Bernard had telephoned a building supply company in London and arranged with the display organisers to allow a truck inside to deliver some heavy material. That's all he told them.

The truck arrived and tipped it's load of building blocks in Bernard's designated display area. Bernard didn't do anything with the untidy heap of blocks. That was his display. He got away with that one!

Memorable were the late evenings in Coaraze, lying in bed and looking down the valley as the light faded, listening to recent popular hits like Procol Harum's *'A Whiter Shade Of Pale'*, played over a loudspeaker somewhere in the village.

Driving from Coaraze to Monte Carlo took about 50 minutes. This was the same road on which Princess Grace of Monaco crashed her car and died in 1982.

There is often confusion about the names Monaco and Monte Carlo. Monte Carlo is one of 3 districts of Monaco, which is a constitutional monarchy.

We stayed with John at Coaraze for a few more days before continuing towards Turkey. At our last evening meal there, with John, Bernard and family, Bernard did something unexpected. Without a word he gripped the edge of the table and leaned forwards, over it, while very slowly pushing himself up into a steady handstand. No wobbling, and very smoothly. Impressive control. There was music playing and everyone stopped talking to watch. Sticks in one's mind!

The following day, the Champ jeep was reloaded with our baggage, consisting of suitcases, bags and even a small fridge. Bernard, no doubt, would be glad his splendid courtyard was free again. We drove back into Monaco and then turned east along the coast, into Italy.

Years later, back in England again, I resumed my contact with John who, by then, was dating Sir Geofroy Tory's daughter Wendy. They later married and everything seemed well. However, John was one day heaving lumps of rock around while landscaping, and had a sudden heart attack from which he died.

John had a profound effect on me. On refection, I see he had influenced me not to slavishly follow social dictates, conventions, rules and expected formalities to the extent one's life lacks character and individuality. The best phrase to describe this is—dare to be different. He certainly did.

REFERENCES/LINKS

[1] *Search: TrojanMuseumTrust.org*

[2] Search: *tankmuseum.org*

[3] Search: *COARAZE The Village of the Sun*

Chapter Seven

ALEXANDER SELKIRK & DANIEL BRUHIN W.

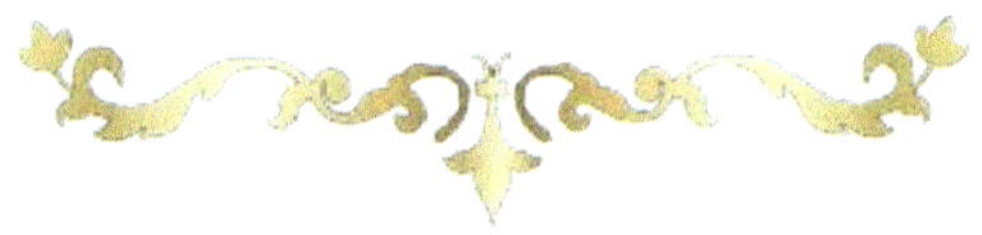

SELKIRK—The Original Robinson Crusoe

DANIEL—Author Photographer Historian

Selkirk (1676-1721)

Daniel (b.1958)

"Solo Robinson Crusoe tiene todo hecho por el viernes."
"Only Robinson Crusoe had everything done by Friday."
Anonymous

OK. So why two names in this title? Shouldn't there only be one name, like the other chapters? Well, maybe not. Read on and you will see why.

Robinson Crusoe. Who has not heard of him? Sadly, fewer and fewer children of the 21stC have. Their parents and all those before them, for 4 hundred years, and living almost anywhere in the world, had heard the story. It was written by Daniel Defoe and first published in 1719. It went on to become one of the most widely published books in history, and even created a new genre—Robinsonade.

And Daniel Bruhin W? The former, Crusoe, is long gone and the latter, Daniel, is alive and well, living in Chile. And I cannot think of one without being reminded of the other, the reasons for which will become clear. So in a way, they are one and the same person to me. My introduction to the story of Crusoe was a book given to me as a birthday present from my brother at the age of 7 or 8. I took to the book immediately. It had pictures that I poured over frequently.

The book was always on hand, never hidden from sight. Inside, were a few hand-written words:

Bryan L. Palmes, Xmas 1912
From his Godfather Hugh E Walker.

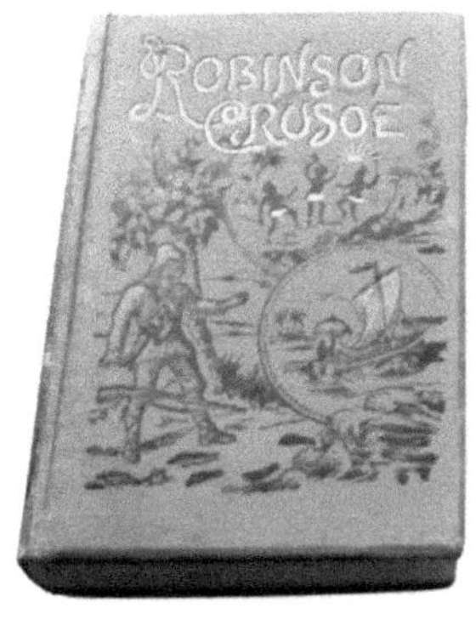

So the book was already old. Under that handwriting I had written my name, saying the book was formerly my brother's. I had written the date I took possession of it—at the age of 10. Why bother saying all this? I think it shows how strong my interest was and still is in this story. Somehow, Crusoe kept my attention, on and off, until half-way through high-school years when I gradually forgot about it. However, both books still have pride of place on my bookshelf.

I don't know where my interest in South America came from. It wasn't the island of Robinson Crusoe as it's location was, in my young mind, never clearly understood. I recall in High School asking the Geography teacher what the next term's subject matter was. She said it would be Australasia.

I said out loud, *"Oh no."*

She asked me what the problem was. I pleaded for her to change it to Latin America, even saying it was far more interesting! She paused and then suggested I think very carefully about what she was about to say. She said she would allow me to study Latin America if I understood that I would get no help or assistance from her while the rest of the class were involved in Australasian studies, and all she could do for me would be to check my intended sources of reference, after which I would be on my own.

I was over the moon. I remember her smiling at my ear-to-ear grin. I thanked her profusely and went on to pass the exam very comfortably. Preston Jame's *'Latin America'*, a tome of a book, was my main reference and I read every page of it. I should praise that teacher's unusual offer. It must have been awkward for her when it came to writing up her records.

Years later, as a young father, I found myself eagerly clambering around rickety ladders and wobbling platforms in a Tudor barn in the south of England. Pure chance and luck had led me there. The barn, owned by a farmer, was jam-packed with books of every shape, size and age. And whatever took your fancy only cost 6 pennies.

Looking back I wish I had bothered to learn more about that massive collection of books, and spend more time there. Anyway, while rummaging through shelf after shelf on platform after platform, I found a book that caught my attention. The ornate compass-like symbol on the hard-cover made me think that something geographical was inside, and I was not disappointed! It turned out to be a 1st Edition published in 1871. It's title was, "Pictures of Travel in Far-Off Lands." I happily handed over my sixpence and have treasured it ever since. A small book of only 11 x 17 cm (4.3x6.7 inches), it nonetheless has 256 pages of riveting first-hand accounts of European travellers to that continent.

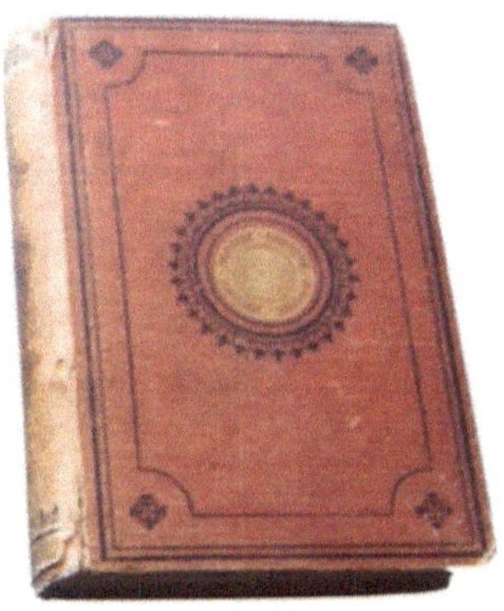

Pictures of Travel in Far-Off Lands 1871
Image by author

It's full title is,*"Pictures of Travel in Far-Off Lands. A Companion to the study of Geography South America"*, published in 1871 by T. Nelson and Sons. It has illustrations of black and white etchings. For me, it couldn't have been a better find, for I was already, I felt, a South American history aficionado. The most interesting first-hand account in the book for me was the section, *'Story of Alexander Selkirk'*[1]. This was my moment of realisation that Robinson Crusoe was very largely based on true facts.

The facts surrounding that island off the coast of Chile where Selkirk was marooned and the birth of the book Robinson Crusoe is as fascinating as anything I have read, and yet is largely unknown. Without giving the subject much thought, practically all people think of Robinson Crusoe as merely a popular fictional account and character. But it is far from being based entirely on fiction. In fact, the real story starts over 400 years ago by a Spanish priest and trader called Juan Fernandez, the discoverer of the little, 3 island archipelago. The following will at first seem like this chapter has gone off course.

Was there ever a place where people were so small they could fit in the palm of your hand? Of course, this is pure fiction. But the setting for Jonathon Swift's "Gulliver's Travels" was not a fictional place as most people imagine. In the early days of European exploration, the first accounts of Western Australia were met with disbelief by people back in England. For example, black swans were described though few people in Europe believed it could be true. But if it was true, they said, it must be the work of the devil because everyone knew that swans should be white! Swift's sarcastic novel "Gulliver's Travels," first published anonymously in 1726 (7 years after Robinson Crusoe was first published), was inspired by two travels to New Holland (Western Australia) by buccaneer William Dampier. Swift even used Dampier's maps of W.A. Briefly, the story is about a man's experience of being a giant in a land of tiny midgets, and then being a midget in a land of giants.

Diana and Michael Preston, joint authors of *"A Pirate of Exquisite Mind - The life of William Dampier"*[2] also ascribe the inspiration for the world's most popular and enduring classics, Gulliver's Travels and Robinson Crusoe, to William Dampier's travel books, themselves born from Dampier's amazing travels.

So William Dampier is the connection between these two famous authors, Swift and Defoe. Having read Dampier's travel stories, Defoe would have found Selkirk's story impelling enough to write Robinson Crusoe at the age of 60. It was his 167th work and his first novel[3] .

Speculatively, Selkirk may have not joined the crews of the 2 ships, the St George and the Cinque Ports, had not Dampier been in overall command on a buccaneering voyage to the South Seas in 1703.

Selkirk had already sailed with Dampier to Western Australia, 80 years before Cook. There is a town named after Dampier on the north-western Australian coast where they made landfall. Dampier had also visited the Galapagos Islands 150 years before Darwin. Though neither Selkirk nor Dampier were easy people to get on with, at least they respected each other's skills. It's likely Selkirk felt Dampier was a reliable 'boss' to go with on a voyage to the South Seas because of his vast and unrivalled experience as a mariner. For example, Dampier was the first person to circumnavigate the world 3 times and was pre-eminent in mapping the winds and currents of the world's oceans. Some of Dampier's observations and measurements are still used today. And Selkirk's skills lay in his navigational expertise. So there would have been mutual respect.

Dampier was the captain of the St George and Captain Stradling captain of the Cinque Ports. Selkirk sailed with Stradling. The journey to South America was full of incidents whereby crew were wounded or killed, and the ships didn't stay together as was originally planned. Reaching the South Seas they separated and Dampier had terrible luck with the St George's almost unrepairable hull. The carpenter plugged the worm holes with a compound of tallow and charcoal because the wood was so rotten it couldn't take any nails needed for a proper repair.

Dampier and his crew had no choice but to sail off in a barque they had captured, after transferring their equipment and gunpowder onto it. Dampier was later arrested at a Dutch settlement because he couldn't produce the required paperwork. He was released after some time and made his way back to England empty-handed.

The Cinque Ports made it to the Juan Fernandez islands. They anchored in Cumberland Bay at the main island, named Mas-a-Tierra by the Chileans, who in 1966 re-named it Isla Robinson Crusoe, no doubt to attract tourists who had made the connection between Selkirk and Robinson Crusoe. For a few days the crew of the Cinque Ports recuperated with fresh food and rest and replenished the ship's stores of fresh water and food supplies.

Alexander Selkirk tried to tell Stradling, the captain, about the serious condition of the ship's hull. It had, in Selkirk's opinion, reached a dangerous state from ship-worm. He told Stradling the ship would probably only last a couple of weeks more of sailing in open seas before sinking.

His next words were the genesis of Robinson Crusoe. He told Stradling he would rather stay on the island than sail with him, to emphasise how serious the condition of the ship's hull really was. But Stradling lost his temper with Selkirk and ordered him and his belongings to be taken ashore immediately. As

Selkirk cried out at the realisation he was going to be marooned, Stradling mocked him, and sailed away as soon as the ship was ready, leaving Selkirk alone on the island.

Stradling set sail for Lima, but Selkirk's prediction came true. The ship did sink with many sailors drowning, while Stradling and the survivors were rescued into captivity by the Spanish. For the next 7 years they were made to work as slaves in the silver mines.

But there is another account about what happened to Stradling and his crew. It describes how Stradling, after marooning Selkirk over the argument, sailed northwards to beyond Guayaquil where they ran aground. On examining the hull they saw it so badly damaged it would not be able to sail again. They surrendered to the Spanish and were taken by an Inca-built road to Lima where they spent the next 3 years in prison, after which they were sent, still as prisoners, to Europe. This account tells of the prisoners being threatened with working in the silver mines if they didn't behave themselves.

It is of interest to mention here something of Selkirk's story up to his marooning on Isla Mas-a-Tierra (Isla Robinson Crusoe). He was the seventh son of a seventh son. In their time, this was of special and significant status in some parts of the world and still is, though less so, today.

As a child his mother treated Alexander as her favourite, expecting his special status to be the making of him. He was a bit of a rebel at school, though he did have outstanding abilities in mathematics, which no doubt helped his later acknowledged navigational skills.

Perhaps there was an inkling of foresight (or second sight!) on Selkirk's part, at the time of his marooning. He felt sure the ship was so unseaworthy it was in danger of sinking. It is also likely the sailors themselves knew the hull was worm-eaten and in poor condition.

Whichever version is the truth, it is certain the survivors' lives after capture were far worse in all respects to Selkirk's 4 years and 4 months on the island alone.

Selkirk did struggle at first. He fell into a deep despair. He realised that he had a great fear—not the fear of starving, but the terror of being left alone on the island. His fear was so great that he did nothing but stay on the beach for months and hope that a ship would come and collect him.

His belongings consisted of a chest containing a few clothes and a quantity of linen, his musket, a half kilo of powder and shot, a hatchet and some tools, a knife, a pewter kettle, a few pounds of tobacco, a Bible, some books on navigation and some mathematical instruments.

While on the beach, most of what he ate was from sea-shells and seals. Eventually, hunger forced him to walk away from the beach and up into the hills to look for other kinds of food. He found greens in the form of edible vegetable leaves and fruit, grown from seeds left by visiting sailors over the years.

The practice of scattering seeds from vegetables and fruits on uninhabited islands was common among pirates who knew that some seeds would survive, providing food the next time they might pass by.

In time all the fresh food and the good climate helped Selkirk improve his health quickly. He began to enjoy his freedom. Rats that had annoyed him at night by nibbling at his toes were dealt with by cats, also left by pirates, along with goats. He befriended a lot of cats by feeding them goats' meat. With so many tamed cats around him at night, the rats soon left him alone. He built himself two huts made of wood from the pimento tree. One hut was a lot larger than the other. This one he made his sleeping room. He stretched some material he had across a home-made, wooden frame to make a bed.

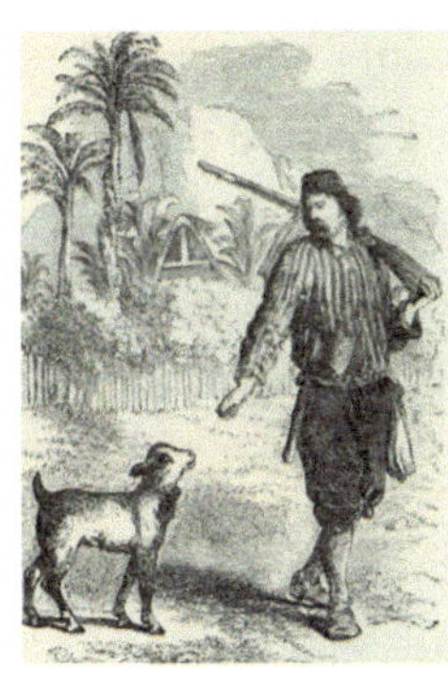

Crusoe with kid goat
Image credits: see[4]

These details of how Selkirk started to establish himself on the island will be familiar to anyone who has read Robinson Crusoe, though the years on the island are vastly different. Selkirk spent 4 years and 4 months on the island, from 1704-1709. Crusoe spent 28 years—which was far better for the plot of a book! Selkirk did become incredibly fit, no doubt because of his natural fresh food diet but also because everywhere on the island seems to be steeply sloping. His method of catching goats (some he tamed), after he used up all his small store of gunpowder, was by running after them. Hence his fitness. Once he fell off a cliff chasing goats and landed on the goat he was chasing, which no doubt saved his life. However, he was so badly injured he lay there for three whole days before crawling and pulling himself back to his huts. His navigational skills told him it had been over three days when he noticed the difference in the lunar phase.

Two British ships ended his solitary existence on the island. They were the Duke and Duchess. Dampier was the pilot of the Duke. The captain was Woodes Rogers, who was impressed by Selkirk's extreme level of fitness and also his peace of mind. He made Selkirk the Duke's second mate.

Selkirk helped the sailors stock up on fresh supplies of food and water. He also went with a few sailors hunting goats. They took dogs with them to help. Selkirk amazed the sailors by outrunning the dogs and afterwards carrying 2 whole goat carcasses across his shoulders all the way back to shore.

Later, Rogers gave him command of a ship they caught, before losing it to the Spanish. Selkirk was then made the sailing master of the Duke. After circumnavigating the world, they arrived off the English coast, making Selkirk's time away 8 years in total.

When finally they disembarked at The Downs, off the East Kent coast, Selkirk became something of a celebrity when he told his story in the drinking dens of London. His share of the Spanish loot had also made him quite rich.

After a most welcome sojourn in London, befriended and admired by so many after such an apparently desolate and lonely 4 years by himself, he travelled north to Scotland to reunite with his family. Largo, the town of his birth and childhood, was reached on a Sunday. He probably had wished for any day other than Sunday because everyone would be at church. Dressed in fine clothes, he entered the church and a few heads turned but no-one seemed to recognise this lost son of Largo. Then, a woman near the front turned her head at this slight distraction behind her. She recognised her son immediately and springing up onto her feet, she called out his name, and ran to him, flinging her arms around him.

There is no record of what the church minister made of this interruption to his service. I hope he was magnanimous though he may have been one of the church hierarchy who more than once reprimanded Selkirk as a boy for his many misdemeanours around Largo.

When it comes to the Robinson Crusoe story, the only arguable point is whether Defoe actually met Selkirk face-to-face in London. And it is doubtful there will ever be any proof found to fully substantiate it. The real point is that Defoe heard about Selkirk's story, directly or indirectly. Already a well-established writer himself, he had Robinson Crusoe published by 1719.

For those who care to study the evidence, there are some very close parallels between Selkirk's account and Crusoe's adventure, though Defoe disguised the location of the island by choosing the Caribbean. Crusoe was not marooned, but shipwrecked and the only survivor. Man Friday was also a fictitious addition to Selkirk's story. After what amounts to only a handful of differences, the similarities between Crusoe and Selkirk are beyond coincidence!

***

I was later to meet up with two descendants of Selkirk and even to hold in my hands Selkirk's drinking cup and examine his sea-chest. The sea chest is held in a warehouse in Leith, the port area of Edinburgh. The Edinburgh Museum gave me permission to view it. To hold Selkirk's drinking cup was quite something. I wanted to keep on holding it! Then later, to examine Selkirk's sea chest, open it and look inside was an electric feeling. In my mind's eye I saw the picture books I had seen as a child, of Crusoe and his sea chest. Total magic!

Sir Walter Scott's interest in Selkirk's drinking cup is well recorded. In 1820 Scott's publisher arranged for the cup to have a stand made of rosewood, together with an engraved silver rim. The cup had been fashioned with a knife by Selkirk from half a coconut shell. It is recorded as having had a silver foot and stem — removed after Selkirk passed away. Probably nefariously.

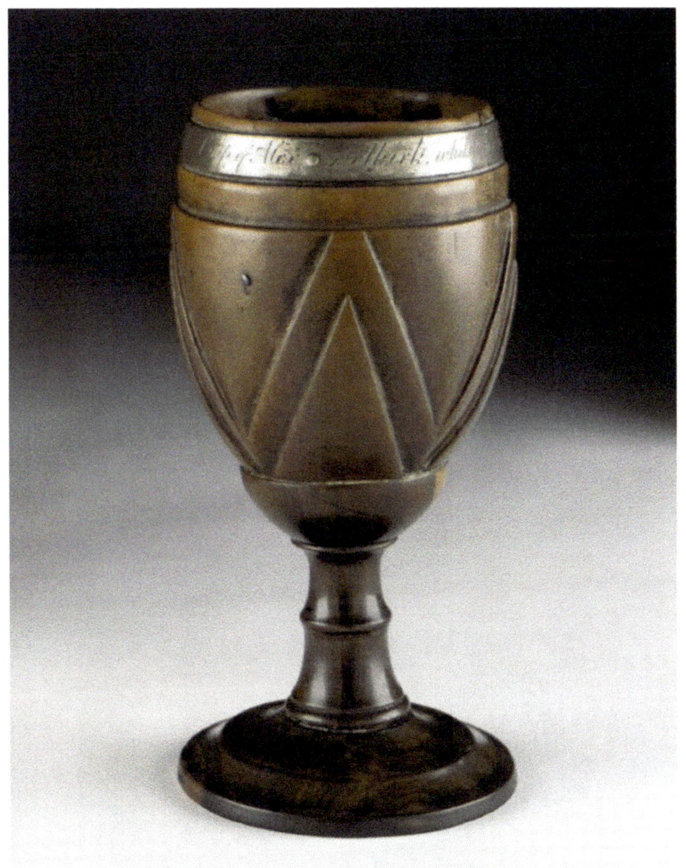

Selkirk's drinking cup

© National Museums Scotland (Permission granted to use image)

The silver band close by the lip of the cup has the following inscription, *"Drinking-Cup of Alex Selkirk whilst in Juan Fernandez, 1704-9."*

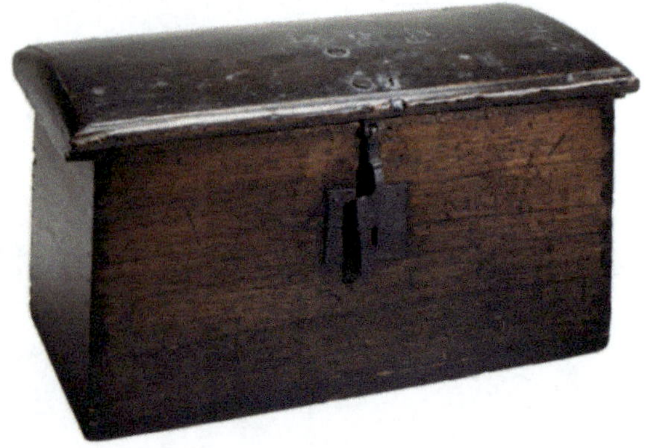

Selkirk's Sea Chest.

© National Museums Scotland
(Permission granted to use image)

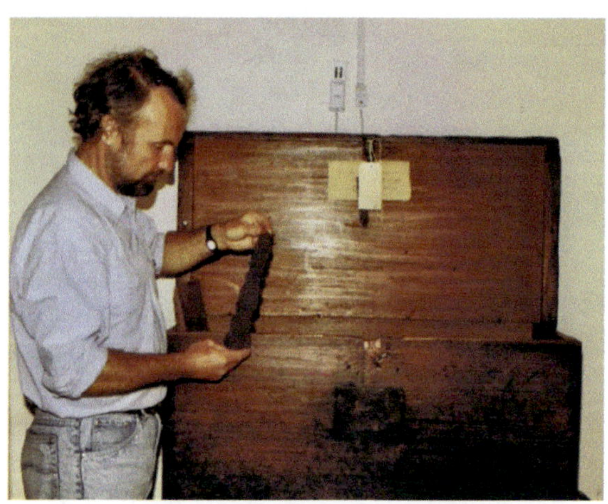

Author examining Selkirk's sea chest

Selkirk's sea chest must be one of the world's most travelled. Before South America and Isla Robinson Crusoe, Selkirk took it with him to Western Australia with William Dampier, 80 years before Capt. Cook reached Australia. Selkirk circumnavigated the world with his rescuer Capt. Woodes Rogers, before reaching England. Selkirk had by then been away for 8 years. The following quotes and image are by kind permission of Dora at *Lundin Links Blog, 2014:*

- *"Selkirk's wooden sea chest and the coconut shell cup are held by the National Museum of Scotland in Edinburgh. They are held in storage and so, sadly, not on public display. Historically, these two articles had remained in Largo, in the possession of the family, even before Selkirk's death in 1721. Catherine Selkirk Gillies, Selkirk's great-grand-niece, zealously guarded the cup and chest according to the North London News of 22 February 1862, until her passing in 1862. She had occupied the cottage in which Alexander had been born and, the article continued .....many visitors had been welcomed to that curious, antique-looking thatched house by its kind old inmate, and had been permitted to drink what pleased them out of the small silver-mounted cocoa nutshell '"*

- *"The sea chest and cup became the property of a Mr James Hutchison of London. Various newspaper reports of late 1863 and early 1864, told his intention was to exhibit the items in London. This idea was short-lived as in 1870 both items were donated to the Museum of Antiquaries of Scotland by linen manufacturer Sir David Baxter of Kilmaron Castle near Cupar. The items had come up at auction and Sir David had purchased them with the express intention to donate them to the museum. The description of the sea chest given at the time of the donation was 'a substantially made chest of teak, 3 feet in length, by about 18 inches in breadth and the same in depth.' The lid is slightly arched above, and closes with an iron tongue or hasp, which comes nearly halfway down the front of the chest, and is there secured by an iron-faced lock. The cup was described as 'formed of a small cocoa nut, 3 and a half inches in depth inside, is ornamented on the outside with a zig-zag pattern. A depressed border runs around the rim in two divisions.'"*

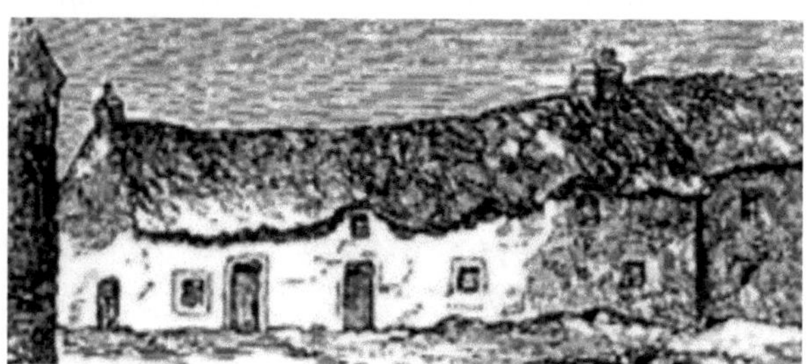

Cottage at Largo in which Selkirk was born. Source: Lundin Links Blog

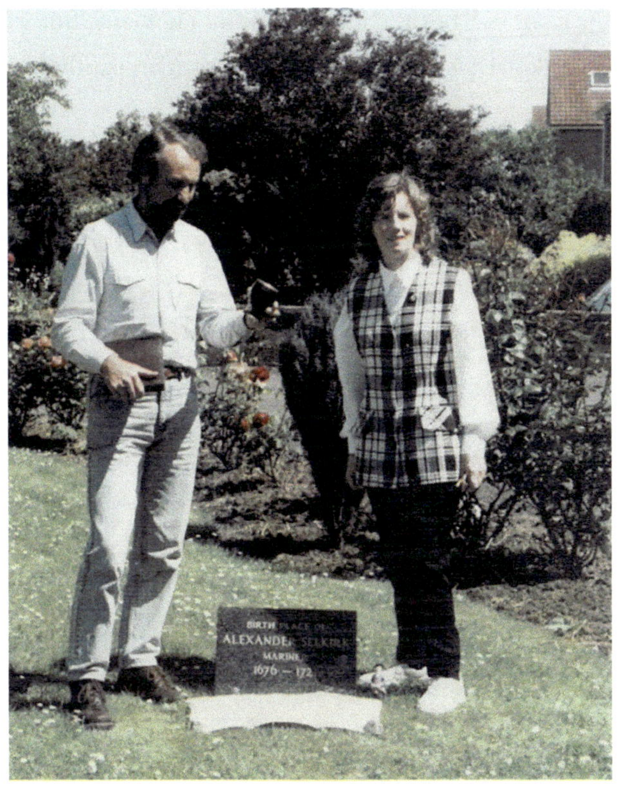

Ivy Jardine, descendant of Selkirk, at home in St Andrews with Selkirk's cup, the Selkirk house title deeds and plaque from Selkirk Museum in Largo.
Image by author, P.A.Brown

After visiting Ivy Jardine and holding Selkirk's cup (before it was kept in National Museums Scotland) I visited Selkirk's home in Lower Largo. It is in a terraced row of cottages. Selkirk's has been altered over the years but undisturbed is a statue placed in the front wall of the cottage, made by Thomas S. Burnett in 1885. Selkirk is wearing his goat-skin attire. A brilliantly detailed statue.

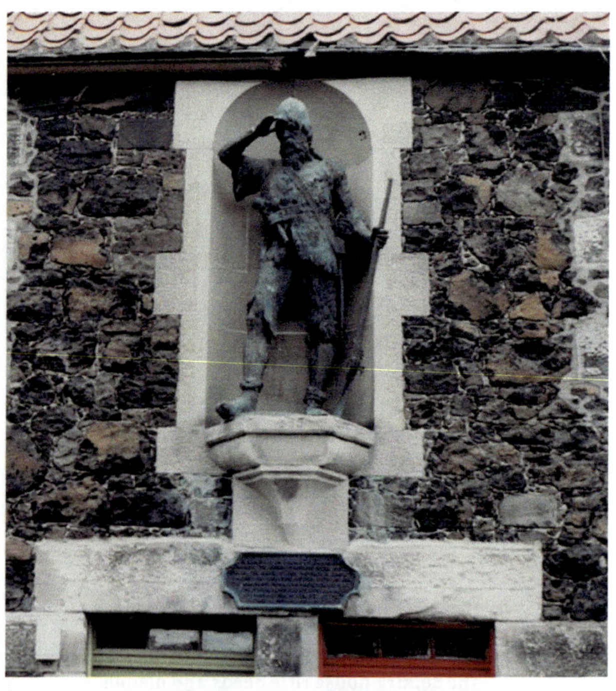

Life-size statue of Selkirk placed in front wall of family home in 1885, made by Thomas S. Burnett.
Image by author

The statue was donated by David Gillies of Cardy House, Lower Largo, a descendant of the Selkirks. The text on the plaque reads:

"In memory of Alexander Selkirk, mariner, the original of Robinson Crusoe who lived on the island of Juan Fernandez in complete solitude for four years and four months. He died 1723 of HMS Weymouth, aged 47 years. This statue is erected by David Gillies, net manufacturer, on the site of the cottage in which Selkirk was born."

The unveiling ceremony was a big affair. There were floral arches over the main streets, with bunting and ever-greens everywhere. At the Crusoe Hotel was an arch with a banner — *"Welcome here the Earl and Countess of Aberdeen."* Some of the other many banners read, *"Weel may the Boatie Row"* - a song with special significance to Largo, *"Robinson Crusoe now we see, good and great at last"*.

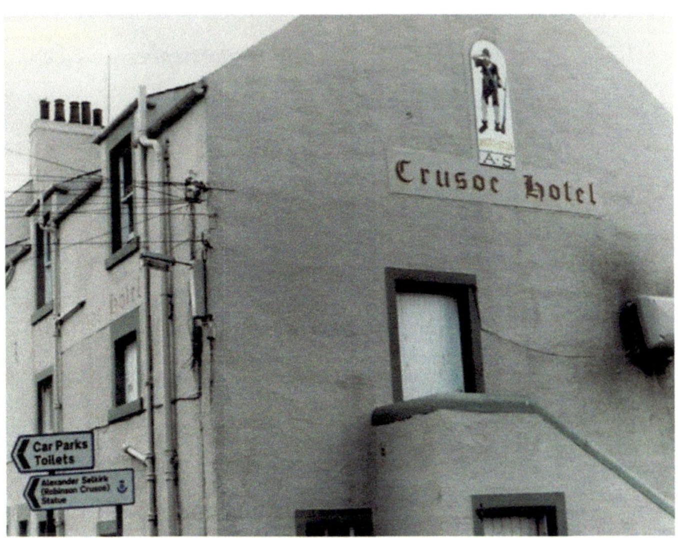

Image by author P.A.Brown

Somehow my fascination with Selkirk was becoming stronger. It had changed from books and articles about Crusoe to tangible artefacts connected with Selkirk. My next thoughts turned to perhaps visiting the island. Should I? Could I?

Fortuitously, in1994, I purchased a copy of Geo Australasia magazine[5] It looked interesting. Imagine my surprise on seeing an article inside—*'Where The Real Robinson Crusoe Was Left To Rot.'* Of course, I already knew where that was.

The article was entertaining though I had a few reservations on some points made by the author, Anthony Perrottet. The photographs, however, were something else. I looked at the first two large photos and being impressed, looked for the name of the photographer. It was Daniel Bruhin W. Imagine my excitement to read at the end of the article;

"Daniel Bruhin W. is a freelance photographer and he has lived on Robinson Crusoe island since 1986."

I immediately took pen and paper and wrote a snail mail to Daniel to say how much Selkirk interested me and that I wanted to travel to the island. Daniel replied my letter and from that day I started planning my first trip to the island.

Once in Chile, there are two ways to reach the island—by boat or plane. Both have issues! The sea off the coast of Valparaiso happens to be where the cold Antarctic ocean currents meet the warm south flowing currents from the north. The result is rough seas pretty much all the time. The Chilean navy travels to the island a few times a year and may transport goods and passengers who reside on the island. Twice a month there is a privately operated supply ship. It carries all kinds of food, including frozen, as well as construction materials, vehicles as well as some local passengers. There isn't much room left for tourists and the cost is high. It takes around 20 hours. It is prudent to have a supply of sea-sickness tablets on hand. It is virtually never calm there.

Occasionally, it is possible to travel by other ships too, though I ran out of luck when I tried that. On one occasion I had arranged to sail by a large boat with the interesting name, *'Charles Darwin'!* I was prevented from sailing on the arranged date because there were unexpected engine repairs needed. I waited 12 days for the ship to sail but each time the sailing date arrived, it was put off for various reasons. I never did get to visit the island on that trip but I resolved to go back some day, which did happen and more than once, but only by air.

Travel by air is the best option unless you love the sea. The flight, though, also has possible issues. It is expensive, and the plane can only be a 12 seater or less because the landing strip on the island is restrictive.

One time I flew there, I sat in the empty seat next to the pilot in the cockpit. After flying almost the whole way of 675 km, the pilot received a call from the island to say it was a no-go. The weather on the island was against flights landing there. So it was a case of banking sharply and travelling the whole way back to

Valparaiso. The family-owned air company upheld my payment and I was able to try again the next day.

Approaching the island's runway is interesting, and if you're sitting next to the pilot, as I was, again, it can be rather alarming. The plane approaches a high, sheer cliff with the runway starting a very small distance from the edge of the cliff. Anyone who has piloted a small plane or done hang-gliding, will appreciate what happens as you approach a cliff edge. There is a tremendous uplift of air that pushes everything upwards. Birds use these updrafts all the time. The pilot therefore has to fly as close to the cliff edge as he can do, to minimise the problem of being able to land at the beginning of the airstrip. And the air-strip is not very long, which is why it is suitable for only small planes.

Another point about travelling there by plane is that you land at the 'wrong' end of the island. The only settlement, San Bautista, lies on the far side of the island and there are no roads going across the mountainous island. You have to travel by a small boat that takes over an hour to arrive. Those sea-sick tablets are useful even if you fly to the island by plane!

My next pleasant surprise was being taken to Daniel's house. It wasn't in the settlement as I expected, but further up the steep slopes and out of sight of the village in what is called Lord Ansen Valley.

We walked a lot, seeing Selkirk's lookout spot high up where it is possible to scan the seas almost 360°. Selkirk often walked up there to search the seas for any ships that may be approaching. And not all ships were welcome. Sometimes a Spanish ship would arrive for the same reason British pirates came—for fresh water and food supplies. Once Selkirk was spotted and chased up into the woods. He quickly climbed a tree and hid in the foliage. The account tells how one Spanish seaman relieved himself at the base of Selkirk's tree. To me that seems a little fanciful but if true, must have caused Selkirk's heart to work overtime.

The habitable part of the island has a beautiful climate with mountains, forests and some unique flora and fauna. Before settlement, there were no snakes nor poisonous spiders. However an exotic poisonous spider was accidentally introduced from the continent. It's bite can be fatal if the patient isn't inoculated with an antidote or flown to the mainland. There is one native species of hummingbird where the appearances of the males and females are quite different, initially leading biologists to believe there were two native species. A second species has since been introduced. They are beautiful to see close up. When exploring a densely wooded valley, hummingbirds hovered within 30cm of my face, checking me out. Some imported trees, eucalyptus being the main example, grow to a prodigious size.

A French colonizer, Desirée Charpentier, introduced the blackberry plant to the island around the year 1910. It must have seemed like a good idea at the time! I have experienced the maniacal size the blackberry plant grows to on Isla Robinson Crusoe. I have described the size of one particular blackberry plant that left many marks on me from its huge thorns, but there is always disbelief in the listener's eyes. In England blackberry grows as a spreading bush, nothing more. This one that 'attacked' me on the island has a trunk, like a tree, of a circumference of about 60-70 cm. Its branches were tree height and its thorns formidable. Eucalyptus trees seem to thrive well here, too. They grow fast and huge.

Once, when walking along the little street of the only settlement on the island, I stopped to listen to a European girl of about 10 years of age, on holiday with, I assumed, her father. She was sitting on a large rock reading aloud to him, while he stood next to her. She read in English a paragraph about Robinson Crusoe who, as Selkirk, had possibly even sat on the same rock. That is a picture I will always keep in my head for being 'literature at its best'.

Selkirk, once he'd returned to his home town of Largo in Scotland, was not comfortable. He used to sit alone on the hillside away from other people, looking out over Largo Bay. He rued the day he was rescued, wishing he could once more be *"... monarch of all I survey"*. William Cowper's immortal first line of his last poem, had tried to imagine what life had been like on the island for Selkirk. But he got it hopelessly wrong, imagining Selkirk was driven to despair. The poem probably reflected Cowper's own tortured mind better than Selkirk's. He suffered from chronic depression, the likely cause of his revered hymns having an overly austere and sombre quality. He had the nickname of Mad Cowper. Still, he is regarded as one of the best early Romantic poets.

Daniel's knowledge of Selkirk is second to none. I was not only impressed but I learned a lot of new things about Selkirk. The quality of Daniel's photography is, in my opinion, also second to none. I've watched him prepare to take a photo. After setting up the camera and lens, making minute adjustments, he waits for the right moment according to cloud movement and sunlight. Occasionally, I worked out I could have had a comfortable snack and a drink while he prepared for a single shot.

Daniel's books are special too. Not only are the books' physical material top quality, the research and writing that goes into them is thorough to the nth degree. One example was his way of dealing with a photocopy of a 140 year old book about Selkirk written by the Rev. H.C. Adams. It fell into his hands in 1991. He resolved to reprint it with corrections and additions from his research as well as including shorter accounts of other castaways on Juan Fernandez island and others. Adding the extra information about other castaways provided a means of comparing the extremes of hardship and loneliness in different places.

Daniel made a suggestion that he may be the reincarnation of Selkirk! Well, if you have read anything about reincarnation, you will appreciate that Daniel's suggestion is not so trivial or flippant as it may seem. The following coincidences are what made him think of it. Bearing in mind he hadn't heard of Selkirk before arriving on the island, the first coincidence is how he learned that Selkirk was aged 28 when he was marooned on the island, the same age as Daniel when he arrived there. Another coincidence is that Selkirk did not see his relatives again until 8 years later; Daniel didn't see his relatives, also in Europe, for 8 years. And yet another coincidence is the land he bought on which to settle and build a house. This happened, as already stated, before he knew of Selkirk, and yet turns out to be the most probable site where Selkirk built his two huts. In looking around Daniel's place over the following few weeks I came to agree with the reasons why this was considered Selkirk's site for his huts. Being there on the same spot where Selkirk had likely lived made it all the more special. What a buzz!

So how have Selkirk and Daniel influenced me? Selkirk proved to me that one's resourcefulness should be tested and skills improved by doing things yourself, if you can. The satisfaction that follows from that is far longer lasting than the items themselves. Selkirk learned to deal with fear and despair. I like to think I could manage that in difficult circumstances. Selkirk also gave me a life-long interest that seems like it will never die which, I only realised on thinking about it, might partly explain why I am never bored.

Until I met Daniel, I didn't broadcast my high and enduring interest in a forgotten sailor of hundreds of years ago. I had never met anyone else who was even remotely interested in Selkirk, even if I made casual mention of him in a conversation. Meeting Daniel with all his connections to Selkirk was more than special. It seemed like a complete vindication of my interest in Selkirk while everyone else seemed to think of it as rather peculiar or merely so-so. If I am reminded of Selkirk for any reason, Daniel is there in my mind too. When Daniel contacts me by email, Selkirk is there too. Inseparable. Quirky? Perhaps, but 'quirky' is often what makes the world interesting and stimulating!

I applaud Daniel for his interest in Selkirk and also because, like Selkirk, he is self-reliant and can turn his hand to whatever is needed. He goes off to very remote and wild places in Patagonia, arguably top of the list of spectacular scenery in the whole world, and spends weeks taking amazing photographs and returning to write amazing books.

Examples of Daniel's photography and books follow:
DANIEL BRUHIN W. - CHILE (South America)

All Photos © 2022 Daniel Bruhin W.
All Rights Reserved

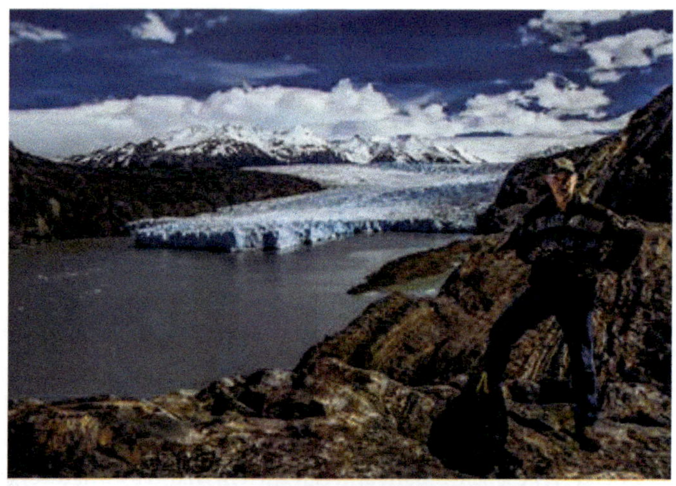

Daniel with Glacier Grey, part of the Southern Ice Field behind him, in the Torres del Paine National Park (November 2017)

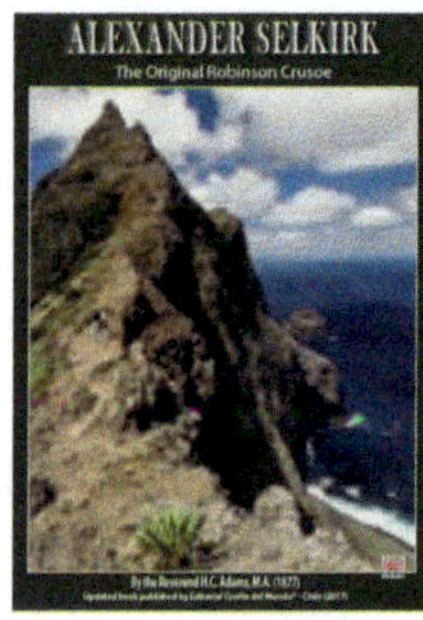

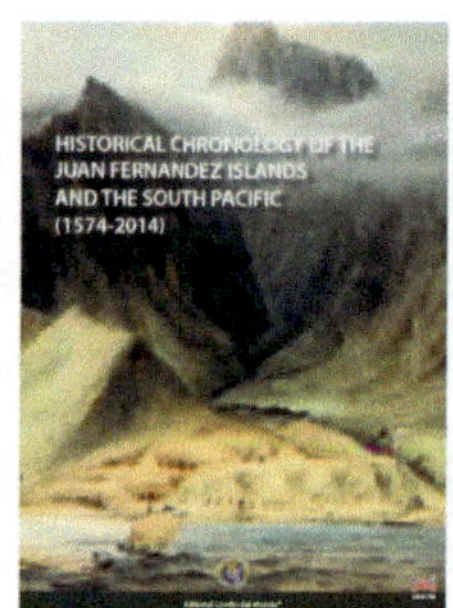

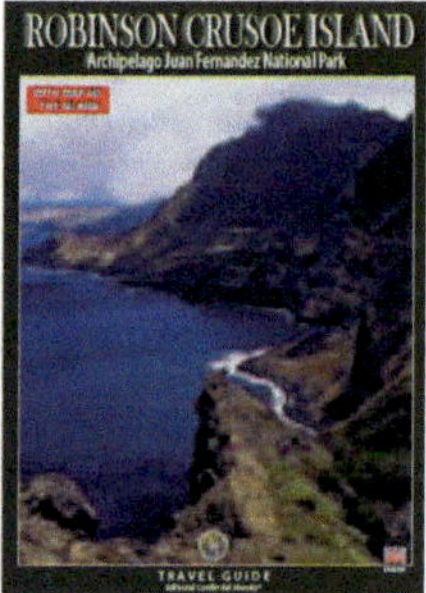

First book on left was published in 2017 in Spanish & English. The other two, as well as a fourth not shown here, are in project. Daniel has also published four other books about Patagonia.

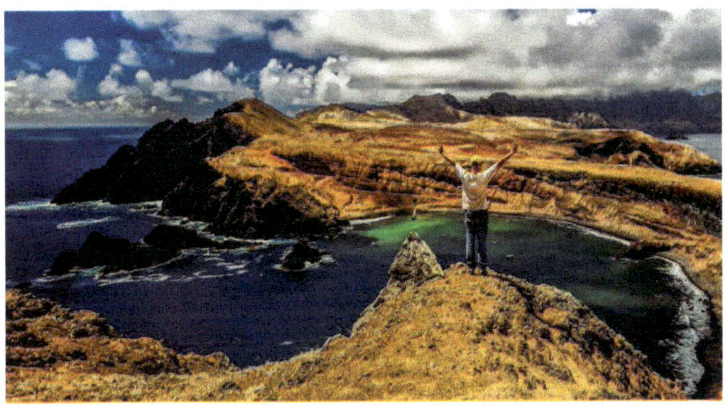

Daniel modelling at south eastern point of the island of Robinson Crusoe, near airport with a panoramic view of the whole island (February 2013)

REFERENCES

1 "Pictures of Travel in Far-Off Lands. A Companion to the study of Geography South America". pub 1871 Nelson & Sons, Edinburgh p 61 Story of Alexander Selkirk

2 "A Pirate of Exquisite Mind. The Life of William Dampier" by Diana & Michael Preston

3 "Robinson Crusoe. The Life and Adventures of Robinson Crusoe"

4 Crusoe with kid goat. Page 70. Pictures of Travel in Far-Off Lands. A Companion to the study of Geography South America", published in 1871 by T. Nelson & Sons.

5 Geo Australasia Volume 15 Number 4, November 1993/January 1994 p106

Chapter Eight

ALAN BROWN

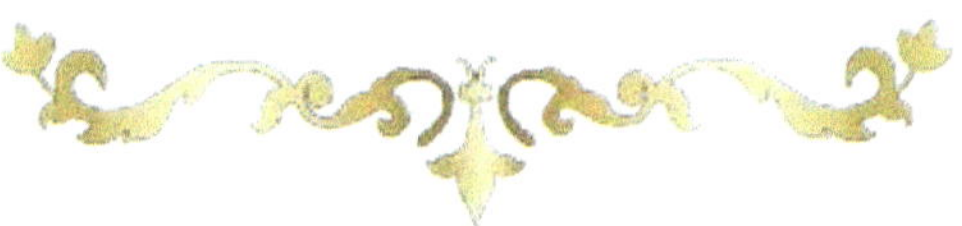

Iron Man of Soccer

(1914-1996)

"One of the truest tests of integrity is its blunt refusal to be compromised." Chinua Achebe

Alan Brown, my uncle, was the first person I was in awe of. As is typical of most British families, our relatives visited, or were visited, now and again rather than often and regularly. Looking back, in those days before computers and personal phones, life seemed a more normal pace compared with today's frantic speed that people seem to think they need to live by. I prefer those older times by far.

As a child all I knew about my uncle Alan was his full involvement with English soccer. His family had children—cousins I barely knew, as the older they got the less they were around when our families occasionally visited each other.

As a youngster I remember a visit by Alan where he left me with a lasting impression. He was describing to my father something that happened a few weeks prior. I listened intently when he mentioned seeing a group of fast moving lights across the sky one evening. That would have been about the mid-fifties when there was a dramatic increase in UFO sightings. My father later told my mother what his brother had said, adding that he must be going 'a bit nuts'. If my father was alive today, he would be reconsidering that remark; the USA is releasing data about UFO's, including film from airforce pilots' cameras, a definite acknowledgement of their existence. Alan's daughter, Angela, told me only recently, that she was in the car with him at the time and saw them herself, too.

My father and Alan were born in Corbridge, County Durham in the north-east corner of England. Their father was a painter and decorator who spent much of his time lying on his back on scaffolding, painting ornate ceilings. The usual practice for preparing the tiny sable brushes for fine details in the pictures was to put the brush bristles into the mouth and get a nice pointy end with saliva. Unfortunately, in those days the poisonous nature of lead in paint was not appreciated. He died in his late 40's from lead poisoning. I had never even met him.

Alan went to Hexham Grammar School, 11 minutes by vehicle from Corbridge. Reading about that school makes me wonder if its tough nature had anything to do with Alan's nick name 'Iron Man'.

In 2021, Brian Tilley, a former student at that Hexham school, wrote an article in the local Hexham Courant paper[1]. He said the school was being demolished and in his opinion some if not most of the former students would not be sorry for its demise. He describes how, as a young boy, being thrust from primary school into, quote, *"... an alien world straight out of a Frank Richards novel, where masters strode round in sinister black robes, first names were never used, and violent retribution was the punishment for the most trivial misdemeanour."*

He went on to describe how the prefects, boys of 16-17, were also authorised to thrash younger boys at their own discretion. Another memory he recalled was a master who carried a large bunch of heavy keys with which he cracked the heads of boys for talking in class, speaking with the local accent or making too many mistakes in their homework. Another master slippered a boy for having a ruler made in Romania! Between slaps of the slipper he chanted, *"I will not have a communist ruler in my classroom."* Today, that sounds like an hilarious Monty Python sketch, though of course not at all amusing for the poor student.

Alan was apparently an outstanding athlete and aspired to becoming a professional soccer player—in spite of his school playing rugby. He played the rugby position *'standoff-half'* for the school on Saturday mornings and *'centre-half'* in football for Corbridge United, in the afternoon. At the end of his school days the Depression prevented any thoughts of university.

Austen Campbell, a cousin, would no doubt have helped inspire Alan to become a professional footballer too. Austen was captain of the Huddersfield Town team and also played for Blackburn Rovers. He played for England, too, in 8 matches between 1928-1931. So it would not have taken much persuasion by Austen for Alan to join the Huddersfield club as a trainee. Alan accepted the offer and hoped that the club would sponsor his further education.

However, things didn't work out that way. He felt he was regarded simply as a member of the ground staff and the club had no interest in sponsoring his study ambitions. Feeling unsettled he left the club and became a policeman for nearly three years.

He eventually left his police job, deciding to try soccer again. The rules however, forced him to rejoin Huddersfield as transfers were not allowed. This time he made good. He put in 57 league appearances before league football was ended in 1939 due to WW2.

So far in his soccer career, then, no real sign of any 'iron man' qualities except perhaps his determination to keep playing. After the war, where he served in the RAF, the transfer rules were relaxed and he was able to effect a transfer from Huddersfield to Burnley in time for the start of the 1946-47 season. Burnley paid Huddersfield £25,000 for Alan's transfer, a club record fee. Time was against him, though, in that he was now 32 years old. Once you reach your 30's in any sport you are regarded as being at or near the end of your career. Fortunately, the Burnley manager saw potential in Alan in spite of his years. It became clear that Alan was a natural leader and before long he was made captain of the Burnley team.

In the first season with Burnley, Alan put into practice his personal ideas of soccer tactics. The main one became known as the 'Iron Curtain Defence'. It must have worked well because Burnley earned promotion from the 2nd Division. They only conceded 29 goals that season which remains a record for a 42-game season. Alan played in every single match.

In the following season Burnley finished 3rd in the 1st Division, with only 1 goal average the difference between Manchester United in 2nd place. It is regarded that Alan's Iron Defence Curtain strategy was integral to their success. Only Arsenal, the champions, conceded fewer goals than Burnley that season.

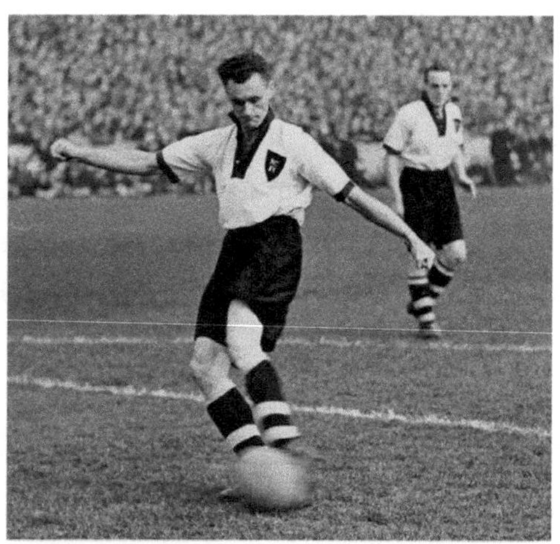

Alan playing for Notts County in 1948-49 season.
Photo: Nottingham Journal Ltd. (merged with Nottingham Guardian in 1953 before closing in 1973).

Then, very early in the next season, Burnley was offered £15,000 for Alan by Notts County. This was a huge sum in those days and, more to the point for Notts County, Alan was now 34 years old. Maybe his age was something to do with his decision to quit after just 3 months and retire from professional soccer.

He moved back to Burnley and started a new venture by opening a restaurant. 2 years later, he was persuaded by Stanley Rous to return to soccer. Rous was the Secretary of the Football Association and later become Sir Stanley Rous CBE and President of FIFA.

So, in 1951 Alan joined Sheffield Wednesday as coach. My guess is that Stanley Rous didn't want to lose Alan's soccer-tactics capability that had become well known. Alan stayed at Sheffield 3½ years then left to begin a managerial pursuit.

In 1954 Alan was back at Burnley as manager. Apparently his return to Burnley was not well received by some senior players because Alan's high moral and integrity values had been increasingly noticed and observed over the years. Ignoring critics, he proceeded to instil his high principals into everything at the club.

He supervised the development of a brand new training centre, employing paid labour and physically helped to dig out the ground himself. He also conscripted some of his players to help out. Jimmy McIlroy was one, probably the most well known in those times. With the help of Bob Lord, the Chairman of the Burnley Football Club, Alan developed a focus on training youngsters at Burnley, which continued long after his departure. During his time as Burnley manager, Alan became recognised for introducing new tactics. He pioneered the use of short-corners and a large variety of free-kick routines, all of which were copied by other clubs.

His managerial time at Burnley was hugely successful. He kept Burnley in the upper half of the 1st Division for three seasons. Maybe at this time of his life, he began allowing in some nostalgia. He was 43 and couldn't resist an opportunity to return to his home territory of Northumberland to manage Sunderland.

However, the club was not in good shape. It was at the bottom of the 1st Division as well as trying to survive a series of corruption scandals involving illegal payments to players. Alan no doubt saw an opportunity to clean up the club.

He once described the endemic practice all over the country of paying young players' parents bribe money to sign up for a particular club. He said on 2 occasions parents had waited until, pen in hand, he was about to sign up their sons and they would say, *"Well, what about a bit of so and so?"*

His reply was, in his own words, *"Look, you can take your boy home if you like, but you won't get anything illegal here."*[2] It took a while for Sunderland to regain its former glory.

At the end of that first season with Alan, the team was relegated to Division 2. It took a few years for the club's performance to turn around and clear out the corruption.

Something I learned about Alan came from being his nephew and listening to conversations when our families met up. He would choose young players before older players and insisted on serious training. He would go with the players to the beach in Sunderland at 6 am weekday mornings. If you know anything about the North Sea, you'll know it's very cold! The players had to have a morning swim before starting training sessions. At times Alan joined them in the morning swims. He was very fit himself and I heard that he once did continuous squat-jumps the whole distance round a full-size soccer pitch without pausing. If you know what squat-jumping feels like, you will appreciate what an amazing feat of endurance that was. That, by itself, shouts *'iron man'!*

Finally, in 1963 the club regained 1st Division and no doubt everyone, fans included, were ecstatic. In the same year Alan dumbfounded the club by quitting at the end of that season.

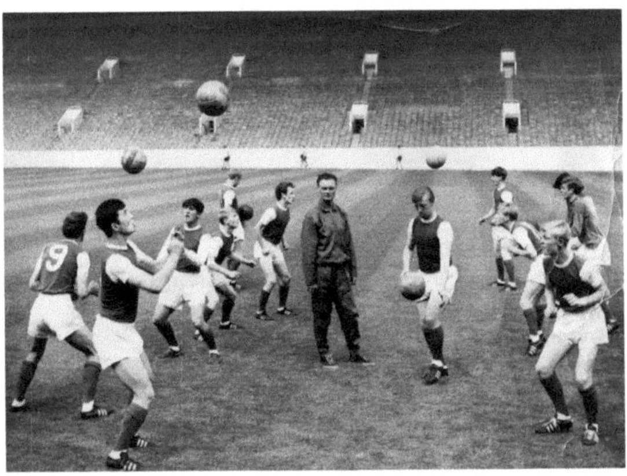

Alan Brown, centre, as coach for Sheffield Wednesday.
Image credited to the former North Yorkshire News Service.

He had been tempted by the board of Sheffield Wednesday. No doubt the board had followed his tough stance on corruption at Sunderland and wanted him to clean up their club following the match fixing scandal. It was called the British Betting Scandal of 1964 in England's association football. 10 professional players were gaoled for offences involving match fixing. This time, Alan was well received and respected by everyone, including players. The club's pride was quickly restored.

In 1966 Alan led the club to the Wembley Cup Final. This was their first final in more than 30 years. The match against Everton was led by Wednesday until Everton made a comeback in the second half and won 3-2. That cup final match is regarded as one of the best finals ever held at the old Wembley stadium. I am sure this must have been the most gratifying part of Alan's football career, though that is my guess only.

In 1968 Alan moved yet again. He returned to Sunderland where the team was relegated a second time. After trying for two more seasons, he was sacked! Not wanting to leave the game altogether, he went to Norway and coached HamKam (abbreviated from Hamarkameratene) at Hamar where he steered the team to finish up second in the Norwegian1st Division, Norway's Premier League.

With good memories of working there, he left in 1974 intending to fully retire from soccer and all the stresses that came with the job of professional football. He went to Bodmin in Cornwall and started a well-earned retirement. Even so, it wasn't long before he received an offer from Plymouth Argyle for the position of Chief Coach. Unable to stop himself, one supposes, he made a successful partnership with Tony Waiters, Plymouth Argyle's manager. Together they led the team to a promotion into Division Two in 1975. Alan stayed with Plymouth Argyle until 1977 when he finally did retire. Supporters and the press in Plymouth tried to persuade him to stay on as manager when Tony Waiters left Argyle. This time, though, he really did fully retire.

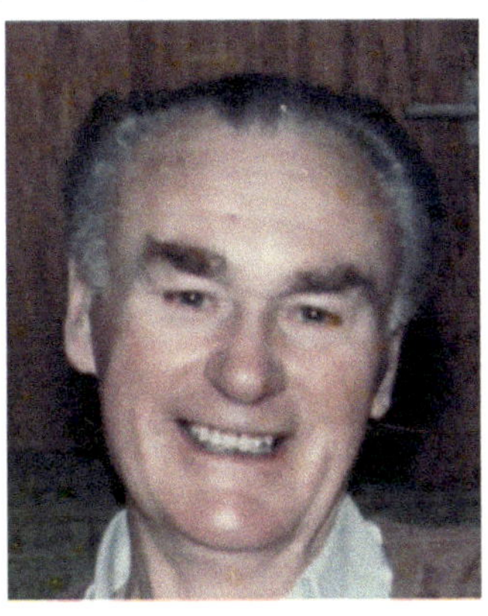

Alan Brown at age 72
Image courtesy of Angela Newsome, daughter of Alan Brown

There's a connection between Alan Brown and Arthur Hopcraft[2], though I have no idea if they ever met. Hopcraft is most likely remembered as a scriptwriter because of his runaway successes like Tinker, Tailor, Soldier, Spy; Bleak House; The Nearly Man; Hard Times; Rebecca. He was regarded as one of the great scriptwriters of his day. Before taking up script writing for TV he was a highly respected sports journalist, working with The Observer and Guardian newspapers. His book, *"The Football Man: People and Passions in Soccer" (1968)* is regarded as a sports book masterpiece. Some even describe it as the best book ever written about sport and still relevant today.

The chapter about Alan is called, *"Alan Brown and Absolute Trust."*[2] In it, he describes how Alan restored public confidence and self-respect at the Sunderland club after the spectacular scandal over illegal payments mentioned earlier. Hopcraft eloquently described how, quote, *"His cold, sorry anger in the face of greed and irregularity in matters of money is one of the institutions of British football."*

Another worthy quote by Hopcraft, *"When Sheffield Wednesday reached the Cup Final under his management in 1966 the players were much aggrieved when Brown absolutely squashed their lobbying for more tickets than the figure laid down by the F.A. as the players' allocation. 'The fact is,' he said, 'that the clubs and the players don't get enough tickets. But the thing to do is to change the rules, not break them. I said I would rather leave my job than break the rule. It was not my business that other clubs would have given way. How does a man manage if he hasn't got courage and responsibility?' "*

Hopcraft noted that while there were many honest men in football, Alan was more fiercely attached to protecting integrity in the game as its central feature. Integrity was, to Alan, more important than brilliance and that success without it is deceit. Halleluja to that.

Iron man indeed, to uphold such strong principles in the face of so much corruption, double-dealing, fraud and cheating.

Think FIFA's scandals in recent years. In 1993, three years before he died, he published a book called, *"Team Coach—Book of Football Coaching."* It contains a list of Alan's proteges—46 international managers, coaches and players who had tuition from him—much to be proud of. His integrity was iron clad, proved again and again.

His title of *Iron Man of Soccer*[3] is most appropriate and worthy.

REFERENCES/LINKS

[1] Search: *Hextol Column: Grammar School demolished*

[2] Search: *Arthur Hopcraft Papers*

[3] Search: independent.co.uk/news/people/ovituary-alan-brown

Chapter Nine

ROSIE SWALE-POPE

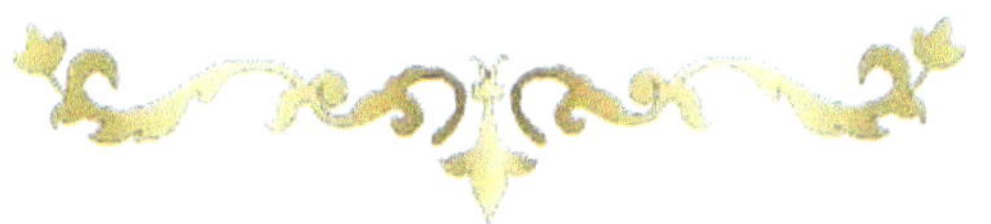

Writer, Adventurer & Ultra-Marathon Runner

(b.1946)

"Nothing is impossible. The word itself says: 'I'm possible!'" Audrey Hepburn

How many people do you know who have ridden horseback for thousands of miles in one go through different climatic zones? How many do you know who have sailed alone in a small cutter (5.2 m) across the Atlantic Ocean? How many people do you know who have run across the Sahara? What about running around the whole world?

None, or hardly any, is the likely answer because they seem such unlikely pursuits or possibilities. But Rosie Swale-Pope has done all those and much more. This chapter will focus on just two of Rosie's adventures for two reasons. One is that if I tried to write about all her adventures, it would take far too long and make up a book in its own right. It would also be out of date as soon as it was published. And besides, Rosie writes her own accounts of her adventures. She is hard to keep up with! The second reason is that I have personal connections with these two particular adventures.

Part 1: Circumnavigation by Catamaran

In 1965 I received a reply from an enquiry I made to Bill O'Brien at the South Coast Catamaran Company, England, about the cost of buying a 30 foot (a little over 9 metres) catamaran. The cash price was £4,975. That was the cost of an average house at the time.I had been feeling restless for an adventure and started reading about catamarans as a safer-than-mono-hull boat for ocean travel. I read of what I thought might be a within-budget catamaran. Basically, for most people, including myself, that quoted price unfortunately meant either a house or a boat but not both. For the following few years there was much thought and hesitation.

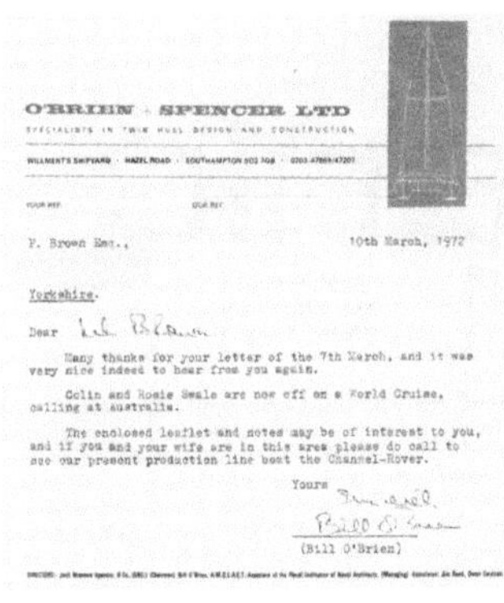

O'BRIEN · SPENCER LTD

SPECIALISTS IN TWIN HULL DESIGN AND CONSTRUCTION

WILLMENTS SHIPYARD · HAZEL ROAD · SOUTHAMPTON SO2 7QB

YOUR REF OUR REF

F. Brown Esq.,

10th March, 1972

Yorkshire.

Dear

Many thanks for your letter of the 7th March, and it was very nice indeed to hear from you again.

Colin and Rosie Swale are now off on a World Cruise, calling at Australia.

The enclosed leaflet and notes may be of interest to you, and if you and your wife are in this area please do call to see our present production line boat the Channel-Rover.

Yours

(Bill O'Brien)

In the summer of 1972 my thoughts returned to the idea of going to sea. I recontacted Bill O'Brien and with my former wife and 2 year old son and baby daughter-on-the-way, drove from Yorkshire down to Willments Shipyard in Woolston, Southampton to meet him. I had read that Bill built his first catamaran at the age of 7, by fixing two pig troughs together! That had impressed me! I vaguely remember reading he was an aircraft designer, whose hobby was building boats. He became increasingly interested in setting up his own boat-building company, which he eventually did, moving to Southampton from Eire.

I was in my early 20's at this time. I remember Bill as a patient, helpful and kind sort of person. He showed me plans and lists of owners of his Oceanic model. I was impressed to hear that all previous owners kept in touch with him and told him stories about interesting happenings while on their 30ft Oceanic yacht. One story he told me about was from a letter received from the West Indies. The owners had been hailed by a patrol boat insisting they abandon their boat immediately and be taken to safety before an imminent hurricane struck. They knew there was going to be bad weather but were unfamiliar with sailing in that part of the world.

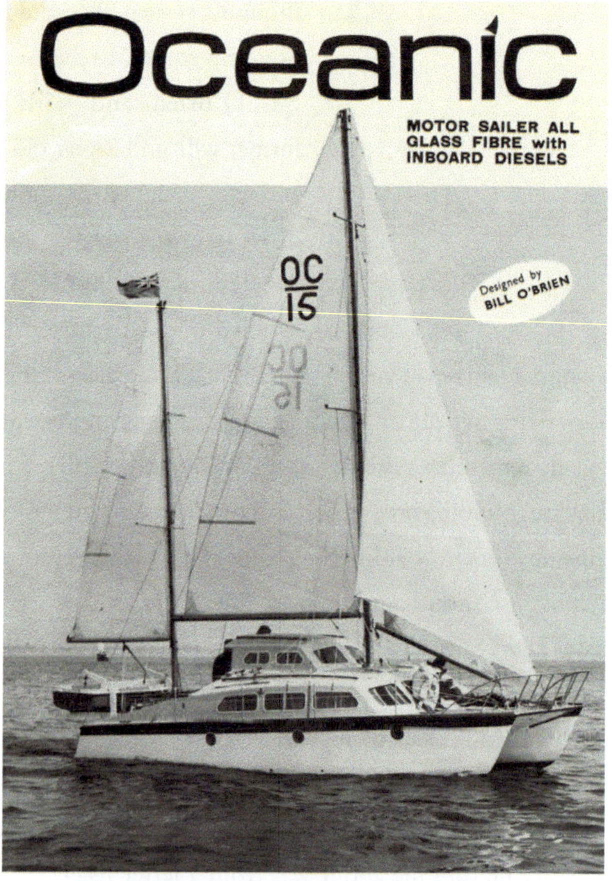

Image: Bill O'Brien's catalogue front cover circa 1965

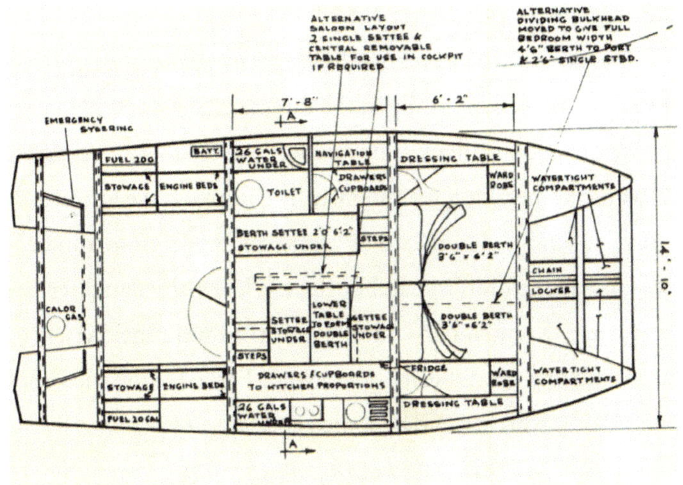

Plan of Oceanic catamaran

Image Bill O'Brien's sales catalogue inside page, circa 1965

They were heartbroken to be forced to leave their boat to the elements and waited for nearly 2 days before being able to go out to search for the wreckage. Amazingly the boat was found with only gouges and scratches over both hulls from being swept backwards and forwards over coral reefs. It was otherwise undamaged. Bill explained that what saved it was the fact of its light weight and small draft. A mono-hull boat would not have survived with its much deeper draft (the distance between the keel and the water level). Bill gave me a list of 35 Oceanic owners dating from 964 to 1970.

He showed us around the small shipyard where he built the Oceanics one at a time. There was a half-finished one there.

I said, *"Oh, a pity it's not more finished, I would have liked to see one with the full deck in place."*

"You can. Go and see the Swales, they have just moved onto their Oceanic," he said, pointing in the direction of a dock.

We drove to the dock and were very excited to see a complete Oceanic in the water, seemingly fully equipped. We introduced ourselves and Colin invited us on board. Rosie, unfortunately, was out so we didn't meet her then. Their baby daughter Eve was there. I remember Colin saying they were inexperienced at sailing and would learn-as-they-go. I asked him when they would be setting sail and he smiled and said, *"Hopefully not long now. We're living on baked beans while we finish buying the rest of the equipment we need."*

Bill also gave me some writing, typed on 2 sheets of foolscap-size paper by Rosie, of exactly that period. Dated 7th January, 1970, it was written only a month after they started living on their boat. She says how almost every day they set off into the Solent with the boat as teacher, and come back a little more educated each time. She describes the boat as being very manoeuvrable and easy to handle under sail. It had two Volvo inboard diesel engines, 3 metres apart, which meant it could turn on a sixpence if needed. A readily appreciated design feature of the Oceanic was it's surprising roominess below deck. Everywhere was above head height so unless you were extremely tall you didn't have to watch your head when moving around. That applied even in the little flush-toilet room with a wash basin. There were two separate double-berth cabins. The large saloon can easily change into extra bunk space, chart room or a dining room.

Their journey of around 30,000 miles (48,280km), took them from Southampton to Gibraltar, Panama Canal, Galapagos Islands, Marquesas Islands, Tahiti, Tonga, Australia (Sydney), New Zealand, Cape Horn, Falkland Islands, Brazil (Recife), and back to Southampton.

They became instant celebrities on account of The Daily Mail writing a serialised account as they travelled. The fact that Colin and Rosie did this with so little initial sailing experience is remarkable enough, but with one baby and then another one being born on board as well, it was even more remarkable. To add to these achievements was perhaps the crowning glory of being the first people to sail a catamaran around Cape Horn, the most treacherous sailing route of the whole world.

I never did try ocean travel on my own boat but I was indelibly impressed by Rosie and Colin's tremendous adventure. Yachting experts had told them it was foolish to try Cape Horn in a flimsy little boat but they were all proved wrong. Their great story became a worldwide bestseller with Rosie's book, *"Children of Cape Horn"*.

Over the years and more adventures, expert opinions and advice were often offered to Rosie, usually with the purpose of dissuading such foolish, dangerous adventures. And always she proved them wrong.

Rosie's next 'impossible' adventure involved going back to Cape Horn, though not by boat. This was to be on horseback from near the top end of the narrowest country in the world, Chile, to Tierra Del Fuego, at the tip of South America.

Equine experts told her it would be unwise to even attempt such a long journey of thousands of miles through such differing climatic extremes.

She did get friendly advice from Major Bill Beldham of RAVC (Royal Army Veterinary Corps). He lent Rosie a special packsaddle, one of only 4 owned by the British Army that was emphasised as being far better than South American pack-saddles which had the reputation of being lethal for horses' backs. The equine experts against her trip-idea told Rosie that no horse could, within a single year, withstand the great heat of the Atacama Desert in the north of Chile and the frozen areas near Cape Horn.

Fortunately, there was an equine expert who did not agree. Only 3 weeks before Rosie's setting off date of July 1984, Señor Germán Claro Lira managed to get word to Rosie, offering to lend her two of his horses. These horses were not just any horses, they were special and unique in the equine world.

Flying to Lima, Peru, from the UK, she then caught a much smaller plane to fly over the border to arrive in Antofagasta in northern Chile. The horses being lent by Señor Germán Claro Lira were still at the hacienda, 1500 km away. They arrived by truck after a few days, and then followed a few days of getting to know the horses and practicing the best way to secure the packs. Aculeo Hornero is a dapple grey—Aculeo Jolgorio a dark bay.

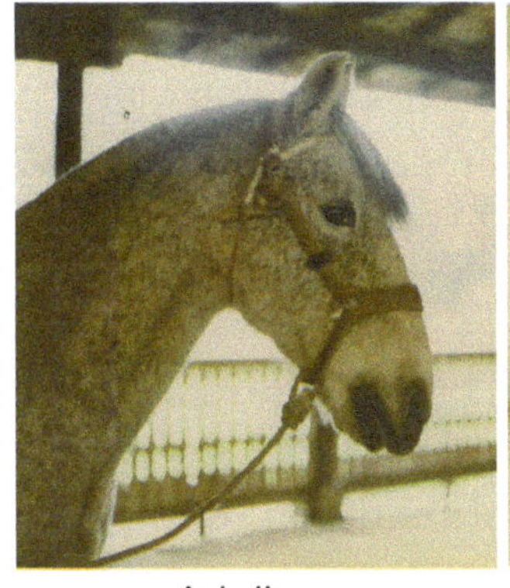

Aculeo Hornero
Image by author

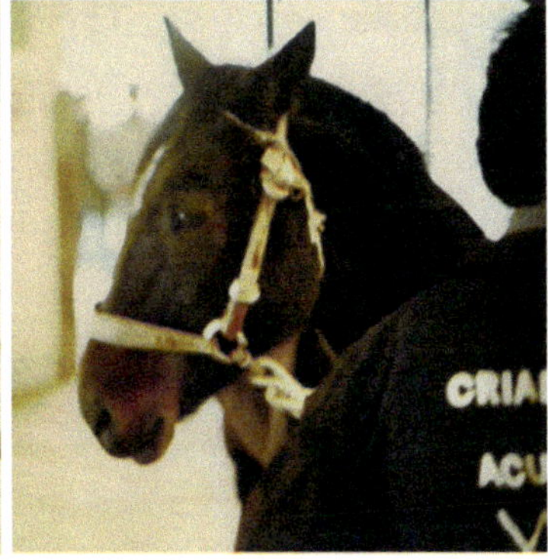

Aculeo Jolgorio
Image by author

Rosie finally set off. I was amazed to learn that one item of her luggage was a typewriter, the same one that she took with her on the voyage round Cape Horn on the catamaran—this being before digital gadgets. The Atacama is not only very hot but also, it is said, the driest place on earth. It is without any plant life and so the horses needed to be somehow continuously supplied with hay and water. Fortunately, the head of the military police was a great horse-lover and he happily arranged for his carabineros to supply hay and water at intervals along the route southwards. Even so, some hay and water had to be carried by the horses. Hay was going to be their only sustenance in the desert, which is not really adequate, nutritionally. During the bitterly cold nights of the desert, Rosie lent the horses her pink leg-warmers and ponchos made up from saddle blankets. I wish there were photographs of this!

One thing Rosie hadn't allowed for almost caused the end to her great adventure. The desert is blindingly hot during the day and very cold at night. If you can put up with that, making sure of hay and water for the horses and one's own food rations, what could possibly go wrong?

Part 2: Back to Cape Horn

Trudging through the sand is simply a question of putting up with the discomfort until you reach a more civilised place. However there was one possibility Rosie hadn't allowed for. A sand storm.

Early one morning, while still asleep, a sudden very strong wind came out of nowhere, enveloping everything and blowing away her tent and any loose equipment and terrifying the horses. Naturally, they were straining at their tethers to run away from the horrible, driving sand-storm. She went to them, tied by their halters to a rope fastened around a large rock. Then, in the panic, the rope snapped and the horses took off. Rosie then needed to protect herself from the sharp, abrasive sand tearing at any exposed skin. Eventually the storm abated and Rosie assessed the damage. The horses were gone, nowhere to be seen. All her equipment was either blown away or buried in sand.

She was most concerned about the horses but didn't even know in which direction they had gone. She mindfully realised if she were to go searching for the horses, she needed something to mark the camp where most of her possessions were, covered by sand. She used a red cotton cloth that had already served many different purposes for a new one that proved critical. She tied it around the rock the horses' rope had been tied to, and set off. It would stand out in the drab yellow sand of the desert when she needed to relocate all the equipment.

She set off, hoping it was the right direction. Later, growing weary in the heat, she noticed she was dizzy and her feet were throbbing. They felt swollen and painful. With a struggle she managed to remove her boots and noticed her heels were bleeding. She had to continue in stockinged feet.

By the late afternoon, after spotting the horses in the distance, she managed a few times to get fairly close, but each time they just galloped off. That must have been frustrating in the extreme. Finally, she managed to touch Hornero and was able to slip the rope she carried over his head. Jolgorio was fairly close by but his halter had caught his hind fetlock and made a nasty rope burn.

With much difficulty she finally made it back to the red cloth tied on the rock and was able to give the horses a little water and some hay she found still trapped in the hay-net. Jolgorio's rope burn was treated. However she couldn't find any of her own food supplies. Nibbling a few strands of hay didn't work.

By now feeling totally exhausted she searched for and found her vitamin supply, mistakenly the veterinary ones. She gave herself an injection of them as instructed by a nurse back home in Wales. Too late she realised her mistake and blacked out. When she came too, in moonlight, she struggled to the tent and sleeping-bag.

The following morning, feeling somewhat better, she organised all the gear and set off westwards. She knew somewhere in that direction was a highway. Eventually, with a feeling of relief, she arrived at the road. Luckily, within a short time, a truck stopped and gave them much needed water and contacted the carabineros who brought with them a vet and a doctor. It was decided Rosie and the horses needed to rest up for a few days in a nearby old mining town. Rosie's journey was anything but plain sailing. Before even completing the desert part she had been considering her attempt to go all the way to Cape Horn an absurdity. Most people would have arrived at the prudent decision to quit. But Rosie is not a quitter, even when the going is extreme. She is immensely stoic.

After more days of 10 hour trekking, the savannah region was reached. Cacti, small bushes, lizards and birds were seen, as well as mosquitos and flies. The horses were no doubt in heaven at their first taste of grass in a long time.

Rosie started from Antofagasta and had now reached La Serena, a distance of 850km by car— possible in 2 long days of continuous driving. Riding across the desert had taken 3 weeks.

I remember being relieved to read that Rosie, while in La Serena, had bought a tape-recorder to replace her type-writer, which no doubt simplified her logbook keeping and significantly lightened her load.

After the necessary rest-up, they resumed travelling south. One late afternoon, Rosie found a perfect camp-site for the night. It was wooded with a little stream. She unpacked and did all the things she didn't usually have time for; washing clothes, bathing in the stream, gathering fodder for the horses and making small repairs. Then a pot of coffee and fried eggs. Everything had turned out wonderful. That night she fell asleep easily, feeling very satisfied and content. But it didn't last long!

Later that night she was woken with the realisation that she and the horses were not alone. There was a rustling in the tight-knit thorny bushes around them. The possibilities were endless, from something innocuous to something terrifying. Human nature usually chooses the latter, so as to be on guard and careful.

It turned out to be a girl, very scared of who might be in the camp. She was also about to give birth. Rosie's camp suddenly became a maternity wing after Jolgorio helped pull her out of the thorny bushes where she was stuck! Having delivered her own second child while sailing around Cape Horn, on board the catamaran, with just her husband and their young child to help, Rosie knew exactly how to help this girl. Everything turned out well and a baby girl was born.

Later, Rosie took them, on horseback, to a village from where the girl had been put on a bus by herself to travel to the nearest hospital, all because the fares were too expensive for anyone to go with her. Being scared and out of her depth with new government regulations insisting all births should now be in hospital with nurses in attendance, the girl had exited the bus long before arriving and tried to walk back home. Instead, she became lost.

The villagers celebrated the birth with a huge fiesta-kind of celebration. They didn't have much in the way of refinements, but they had overflowing generosity and kindness. Their houses were just wooden shacks, though their gardens were bursting with fruit and vegetables. Hornerio and Jolgorio were included in the celebrations, of course, and the children put garlands of flowers on them while they ate piles of carrots and cabbage leaves. The new baby was christened Rosita Angelica Lopez, Rosie for short!

Continuing southwards, Rosie avoided the sprawling capital city of Santiago and headed for the south end of the central valley where stood Hacienda Los Lingues, Jolgorio and Hornero's home. She was accompanied by two huasos, sent to escort her to the family home where a reception was being arranged.

Arriving, the horses were taken to their own stables and groomed and pampered while Rosie tried to adjust from rough camping in a very dirty tent and clothes, to a Relais Chateau standard environment. Her tent was cleaned and erected in a garden so that it and the horses could be photographed by the media. The visitors, apart from the press, were mostly dignitaries such as the British Ambassador and his wife, the Minister of Education, the French Ambassador, and Margarita Ducci, a famous architect, and a whole bunch of Santiago socialites.

After the celebrations, the vet who had known the two horses since their birth, checked them over to make sure they were ready for the next stage of the long journey. All was good except for Jolgorio's hind hooves which were badly worn on their front edges. So, for the next two weeks or so the horses continued to be spoiled, allowing Jolgorio's hooves to grow back a bit. While enjoying the luxurious lifestyle and welcome rest, Rosie was fidgeting to resume the long ride, but Jolgorio's hooves were slow to grow. Eventually the vet gave the all clear.

Once more Rosie and the horses set off southwards. This time the people of the villages and towns she passed through knew who she was due to the publicity from the media at the hacienda celebrations. It wasn't all skittles and roses, however. Rosie broke some ribs falling from a balancing act on Hornero's back. Hornero had never seen a train before, and Rosie hadn't even noticed the tracks nearby. And the train driver was so impressed with Rosie's act he had hooted the train's loud horn to which Hornero bolted and Rosie crashed awkwardly down on the hard ground. There were multiple broken ribs and other issues. It took a few more weeks before Rosie could even think about resuming her journey.

The day after Rosie's accident, 25 carabineros' cars blew up with some deaths, not far from where she was recovering. This was the work of a left-wing terrorist group. A curfew followed. After many weeks of recuperating she was able to set off once more, albeit still in much pain. She encountered many unexpected situations and received much generous hospitality from those she met. The landscape and climate changed. The roaring 40's lived up to its name. The topography was increasingly erratic and bewildering—dense forests, mountains, inlets and islands. One memorable storm that hit in the middle of the night took away her tent and resulted in her sleeping bag becoming a soaking sponge. Knowing that in these latitudes in southern Chile, it can rain almost every single day of the year, Rosie had to accept the fact that daily life would be even more difficult, and wet.

One night she had an unforgettable visitor. A puma. No doubt it thought the open tent offered a cosy change to the weather outside. It must have been unaware of Rosie's presence hidden inside the sleeping bag. But when she couldn't hold still any more and moved slightly, the puma sprang up in surprise and bolted. Further south she had to get used to leeches that somehow managed to find their way into her sleeping bag at night.

Then Hornero got an infection in a hoof from an old man with some shoeing experience, but, as it turned out, not enough. A wrong nail hole into the shoe caused a serious infection that proved very difficult to deal with. It caused Hornero to limp in pain. Vets and horse-people thought the best thing was to euthanise the horse and just get another. That, of course, was out of the question for Rosie.

She finally made it to Cape Horn. It had taken 409 days to late August 1985. She then returned the horses to Hacienda Los Lingues. Shortly after that at the beginning of September, she visited the lighthouse on Cape Horn and signed the logbook, including the names of the horses. She described this expedition as the hardest one yet, and only her obstinate instinct had kept her going.

Because the Aculeo Stables at Los Lingues are so distinctive and have such a long and fascinating history, before continuing it is worth painting a picture of just how special the whole hacienda set-up is, describing the origins of this most distinctive and valued breed of horse, the Aculeo, the qualities of which allowed Rosie's extreme journey.

Part 3: Hacienda Los Lingues

To the casual observer from abroad, Chile rarely conjures up more than a political nightmare. To those who have travelled there, it is a country with the widest variety of climate and scenery. The part played by the horse in its European overthrow, along with the rest of Latin America, was uppermost.

Begun in 1537 by Spanish Conquistador Diego de Almagro and three years later by Pedro de Valdivia, the story of the traumatic birth of this new extension of Spain is littered with gripping accounts of hardship and heroism. Against this kind of background, it is unsurprising that something exceptional would appear. And it did, in the form of a unique breed of horse.

Loosely speaking, the Criollo is the basic Central and South American breed—descended from the Conquistadors' war horses—with variations occurring from country to country. The original blood stock was Andalusian, Barb and Arab. The Criollo's hardiness and smaller size of 13.3 to 15 hh is attributed to the extremes of climate and terrain and natural selection over hundreds of years. (hh = hands high, where 1 hand is 4 inches. The measurement is taken from the ground to the horse's withers)

Hacienda Los Lingues is the only stud in the world to produce the pure bred Aculeo (or Aqualaos) horse. This Aculeo 'version' of the South American Criolla, or Caballo Chileno, is the most selectively bred of South American horses, and in the whole of the Americas is second only in its long and meticulous breeding history to the Paso Fino of Puerto Rico. But while the

Paso Fino is true to the original Conquistador horse, the Aculeo is developed from it. Selective breeding began in 1760.

It will surprise some that the famous Lippizaner of the Vienna Riding School was bred partly from Aculeo lines. Señor Germán Claro Lira, owner of Los Lingues, is rightly proud of the reputation of the Aculeo horse. Used in the War of the Pacific in the Atacama Desert, the Boer War and the Crimean War, it is often the first choice where toughness, endurance and reliability are main considerations.

Los Lingues is located 120 km south of Santiago, in the Central Valley. This part of Chile is described by the South American Handbook as, *"One of the world's most fruitful and beautiful countrysides...."*

Unsurprisingly, most of the country's population lives here, enjoying a climate not unlike Perth of Western Australia, a Mediterranean climate with winter rain and dry summers. The latitude is the same as Perth and the South West, though an obvious contrast with Western Australia is the presence of the Andes rising in Chile to nearly 7000 metres.

Part of the Angostura estate, the hacienda was a gift from the King Of Spain to Melchor Jufré del Aguila, a writer and mayor of Santiago, in 1545. Later the property was inherited by his daughter Ana Maria del Aguila, from where the Claro Liras came. This makes its present keeper, Señor Germán Claro Lira, owner of the longest held family seat in the whole of the Americas, north and south. His wife, Lady Maria Elena from the Lyon family, is descended from Lord Glamis of Scotland and the Earls of Strathmore, and therefore related to the British Queen Mother (deceased).

The stables are unique in their own way. Germán rented a quarry which enabled him to lay 3500 square metres of pink marble for the floors. The stalls are made from thick hardwood with roofs of pantiles like the rest of the hacienda, and most are open and airy. There are horse baths, a delivery room and a laboratory. Special attention is given to morphology and blood lines, the intention always to produce a horse that is strong, resistant to disease and adaptable to any climatic conditions. Until ready for breaking, foals are sent to the nearby Andean foothills to develop their muscles.

A veterinary visits once or twice a week to check the horses. Artificial insemination has not been permitted to date, though in a long distance market with an approved representative, Germán is open to the possibility. The horses begin their training at two and half years with cinch strap and rider. One could be forgiven for assuming it wasn't the first rider or piece of harness because the horse doesn't show any nerves or apprehension. This is when newcomers can see for themselves another hallmark of the Aculeo—a distinctly calm disposition.Their apparent lack of nerves makes them especially suitable for children.

The horse is almost rideable after this first session. The whole breaking process takes around eight weeks. Once broken they are ridden daily except when lunged. This takes place in *"The Garden of a Thousand Roses"* with a fixed rein on a revolving pole. A fully trained Aculeo will have passed tests including the following: galloping to an abrupt stop which causes the hind legs to slip between the forelegs into almost a sitting position; turning on the gallop on one foreleg while continuing to gallop; the same but more difficult manoeuvre on a hind leg; the figure of eight canter in less than a ten metre stretch; turning on the spot through swivelling on one hind leg and galloping off in the opposite direction.

Those responsible for breaking and training are the huasos (cowboys). They live on the estate or close by in the nearby town of San Fernando. It is common for generations of the same family to have lived and worked here.

Besides the breeding and training of horses, fruit growing is an important part of the estate's economics. In high season there are up to 350 workers collecting pears, grapes, plums, apples and berries for export. The huasos and their families have in some cases been connected with the estate for up to ten generations. Some have moved on only to return later.

Families are given a house, health cover, a plot of land to work for themselves, free water, free primary education and, depending on the number of children, a quota of animals they can freely trade.

The hacienda operates as a showplace for the Aculeo and so regularly there is a full blown rodeo, a sport so popular in Chile it is second only to soccer in popularity. One unusual feature is the stopping of a cow by two riders without the use of ropes. One horse 'chests' the cow to a stop while the other rides close behind to prevent the cow turning. The rodeo takes place in a large arena called the Media Luna (half moon), constructed of a high, outwardly sloping, solid timber fence.

Although geared for tourists, Señor German makes it clear that the hacienda, especially the horse stud, is not a set-up for tourists. Since 1980 he has opened the estate to the public to show how a traditional Chilean hacienda and horse stud operates. Visitors can arrange to have lessons in riding, request a rodeo and lodge in the beautifully appointed period rooms. The horse stud, then, is only one of many attractions for visitors. The hacienda can be said to be in a class of its own.

An additional reason for horse-loving tourists from around the world to visit Los Lingues is Rosie's 1985 book, popular in literary circles, of her epic ride to Cape Horn on these two Aculeo horses, not to mention the publicity and television chat shows about it.

The extraordinary situations they experienced make Rosie's book a fascinating read full of surprises. The two horses, Hornero and Jolgorio, have been enjoying a well-earned retirement for many years. They are often the reason for visitors finding their way to Hacienda Los Lingues.

While Los Lingues continues its meticulous breeding program, Aculeons are exported to Holland and Spain, with some sales to Italy. Señor Germán was keen to attract an Australian buyer at the time I visited, to introduce the breed there. A special place in many ways, Los Lingues has become a Chilean institution, a masterpiece, and an increasingly popular tourist destination.

Part 4: A later view of Hacienda Los Lingues

In 1997, years after Rosie's amazing journey on horse-back, I arranged to travel to South America which was to include a visit to the hacienda and hopefully meet those two horses.4 weeks before setting off from Australia, I had a thought. I wrote a letter to Rosie via her publishers. Two weeks before I left there was a reply, wishing me well and that I would get to meet the two horses. She also gave me the address of an elderly lady in Viña del Mar, Anita, who had just translated her book into Spanish.

On arriving in Santiago I went to the hacienda's office to arrange a visit to Los Lingues in a few days time. With some free time, I wanted to see the port city of Valparaiso, an hour's travelling time from Santiago. This was also the opportunity to visit Rosie's friend Anita. Viña is only a 10 minute drive from Valparaiso.

I ended up visiting Anita for three days running. A young 85 years old, she showed me her translation of Rosie's book, took me around Valparaiso and introduced me to Carlos Helvez who had arranged the horses for Rosie's ride. He had been featured in the book and so was all the more interesting to meet.

Since the ride, when Carlos was a journalist, he had ventured into politics. Failing his first election he had gone into managing a University's recreation and media programs. He had then married a Russian girl who disclosed she was relieved to have been born on the right side of the Caucus Mts and so considered herself a European Russian.

Carlos gave me some copies of newspaper articles on Rosie's ride and two copies of his political platform profile, complete with its 'trust me' photos, one for me and one for Rosie. I'd told him I intended seeing her in Wales if she had returned from her trek alone across Albania, where she was at that moment. Of course, Rosie wasn't just sitting at home in Wales!

A few days later my arranged visit to the hacienda came. The weather couldn't have been worse. The 1hr 40 minutes trip southwards by bus was beset by strong winds, torrential rain and flooded roads. Tree branches swept onto the road had to be avoided by the driver. Up in the close-by Andes much damage was caused in some villages. On arrival at Hacienda Los Lingues I was led to a huge verandah on the front of the house. There were some plain old wooden and very long benches, 125 years old, made by local Indians. I estimated there was space enough to seat about 70 people or more on this verandah alone! Going inside, by comparison, were extremely ornate, carved benches, also made by Peruvian Indians. In the entrance hall was a very grand and ornate 17th century French mirror, the largest of its period in the world.

Lady Marie Elena greeted me with hot red wine. A pleasant conversation followed and while talking I noticed a few framed photographs of Rosie, who then became the topic of conversation. I said I had exchanged mail with Rosie about visiting the hacienda to see Jolgorio and Hornero and mentioned my association with the Oceanic Catamaran. Lady Elena suggested waiting till the morning to see the horses because of the atrocious weather.

She showed me part of the hacienda. It is full of unique and priceless treasures from all over the world, including an equestrian museum of much diversity and interest. There are surprises at every turn. In the family chapel, adjacent to the stables, is a large ivory Christ with skull and crossbones that belonged to Pope Pius IX. Its sculptor is believed to be Benvenuto Cellini. Apparently there are very few statutes remaining of Christ with a skull and crossbones at his feet.

In the early evening I was treated to a very grand dinner which would have been attended by, had the weather not been so atrocious, the Australian Ambassador and his wife. Other guests too had elected not to come because of the bad weather. So I got all the attention! Lady Elena, her husband and other members of the family attended. We were waited on by three male servants dressed in white uniforms. A very impressive antique silver service graced the centre of the huge, long table while log fires roared away at both ends of the dining room.

After the meal the rain had somewhat subsided and I was shown over more of the hacienda. As a member of the Relais & Chateaux exclusive hotel group, I was viewing accommodation at its best, which I was able to experience that night, in a most luxurious and beautiful room. The period rooms are authentic in every detail, including not just the furniture but also the wallpaper and plumbing!

The next morning I met the 2 horses that Rosie had ridden that immense distance. Aculeo Hornero and Aculeo Jolgorio were lovely to meet. In a strange way, it felt like meeting two equine dignitaries, if that can be said. Then they were led back to their paddock.

Later, I asked Lady Elena a favour. An idea had been forming in my mind when I had met the horses, close up. I asked if I may have some of Hornero and Jolgorio's hoof clippings. She asked me what on earth for. I told her that I wanted to have a pair of silver earrings made with small pieces of hoof for Rosie.

She paused then said, *"On one condition. That you make a pair for me too."*

I agreed and she took me outside and called for the horses to be brought into the yard. Only Jolgorio appeared because Hornero had shoes. I was allowed to pick up one of Jolgorio's hoofs and see for myself how they were. I think the farrier standing nearby was pleased I knew how to raise a horse's hoof without being kicked. I'd had practice.

Some pieces of Jolgorio's hooves were trimmed off and handed to me. I promised to send the earrings as soon as I was able. I put the pieces of hoof into a small plastic bag but quickly realised one bag was not enough. The unpleasant smell, not unlike the worst sweaty human feet you have ever smelled, resulted in 4 plastic bags inside each other.

I thanked Lady Elena and she took me again into the equestrian museum to look at things in more detail. Not to be totally outdone by this wonderful display, I pulled out of my pocket something I had carried with me for over twenty years. It was a metal clasp I had found at the side of a sarcophagus, near Izmir in Turkey. I had never had it authenticated, but it looked so very old with its beautiful horse-head emblem. I offered Elena this clasp because here, I ventured, it would be seen by many people, whereas in all the years I had kept it, very few saw it.

Later, Señor Germán's sons examined it closely. The next morning Elena showed me where they had put it. Already it was in its own little, blue, velvet-lined box in a large glass case among silver spurs, saddlery pieces and other equine items.

Before I left the hacienda, Elena's brother gave me a beautiful thick, heavy, hand-made, red, black and grey poncho, the kind worn by huasos in all weathers, including downpours. Then it was my time to go. I was offered a lift into San Fernando and I gratefully accepted as it was teeming down again. I put my gear in the boot of an incredibly muddy car, as if thick mud had been poured all over it.

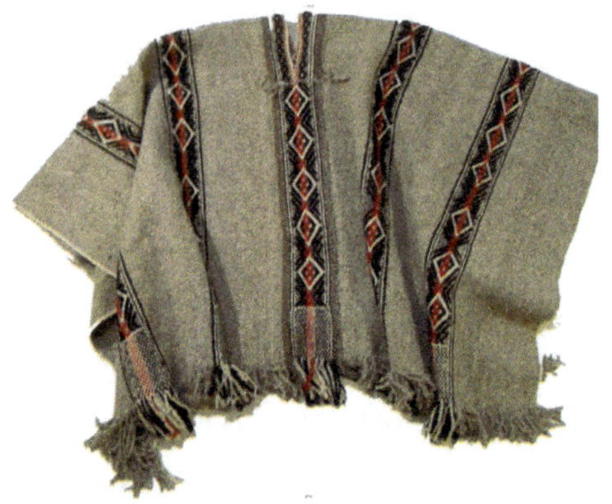

Chilean huaso's heavy poncho given to the author by Señor Germán Claro Lira and family at Hacienda Los Lingues.
Image copyright— author

The speed at which we drove caused huge walls of reddish brown, thick mud to fly in all directions including covering the windscreen for brief moments between swipes of the wipers. It was exhilarating if not unnerving.

By the time I arrived in Santiago the weather was brightening up. Over the next few evenings I repeatedly cleaned and split the pieces of hoof along any cracks I could see. Eventually I had pieces without any visible cracks and the smell was gone. I started making enquiries about local silversmiths. The University of Santiago, one of the oldest universities in Chile, had two students who made items from Chilean silver using the centrifugal casting method. That implies using an articulated arm spinning freely around a vertical axis, though the two students had none of that machinery. Instead they spun their molten silver in little moulds at arm's length, tied to the end of a long thin string.

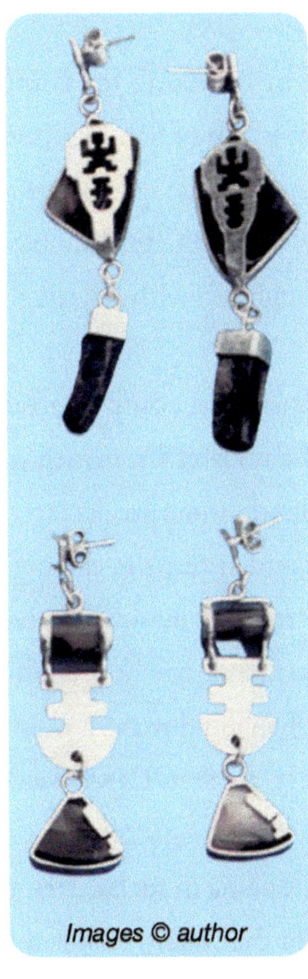
Images © author

I introduced myself and asked if they would be willing to make two pairs of earrings from silver and horse hoof clippings. They were intrigued with the idea, though doubted horse hoof would be a suitable medium to work with. I showed them the pieces and they examined them minutely, checking I think, the hardness. They polished one of the larger bits and started smiling at the effect it produced. They asked if they could make them in an Inca design to which I readily agreed.

Paying them in advance, we shook hands. I gave them an address in England to send them as that's where I would be in a few weeks time when the earrings were ready to post.

Determined to see something of the Chilean Andes, I decided to travel north. I caught a well-appointed coach that impressed me with just about everything plus a few unexpected things. People smiled a lot. I saw the sharing of snack food and fruit. It was very comfortable and clean. And best of all was the singing conductor. He walked slowly a little way down from the front and turned to go back to the front, all the while singing in a very good baritone.

The atrocious weather was part of my thinking for going north. I went first to La Serena, 473 km north of Santiago and capital of the so called IV Region of Chile. It is a delightful town to visit with neo-colonial buildings and about thirty churches. A loud chiming clock rang dully as I caught up with my rough and ready travel notes.

La Serena was one of the places Rosie had come to after riding through the desert. A couple of days later I returned to Santiago to arrange my flight to England. Some weeks later, in England while visiting my mother and sister, the earrings arrived. I travelled to Tenby, in Wales, to meet Rosie and give her one of the pairs of earrings, allowing her to choose. She was delighted with them and told me she would make a point of wearing them whenever she gave her *'Back to Cape Horn'* motivational talks.

I have wondered just what keeps Rosie going in such extreme conditions and happenings. I am certain that many people die thinking that they could have had so many more life experiences had they thrown caution to the wind, at least a few times. Then they would have deep memories to look back on.

While I was in Chile she was riding a horse alone across Albania where at one point she was taken captive by a bunch of brigands and held for a few days before being set free.

Perhaps Rosie gets her dogged determination from words like this;

"If you think adventure is dangerous, try routine, it's deadly." Paulo Coelho de Souza

To illustrate how Rosie never stops, this extract from her 2022 webpage[2] shows how impossible it is to keep up with her!

"Now, at the age of 74, Rosie has taken on an exciting, new challenge: a run of 6,000 miles from Brighton all the way to Kathmandu in Nepal in support of PHASE Worldwide."

REFERENCES/LINKS

[1] Rosie's book and many articles: Search: *'Back to Cape Horn'*

[2] Rosie's webpage: *rosieswalepope.co.uk*

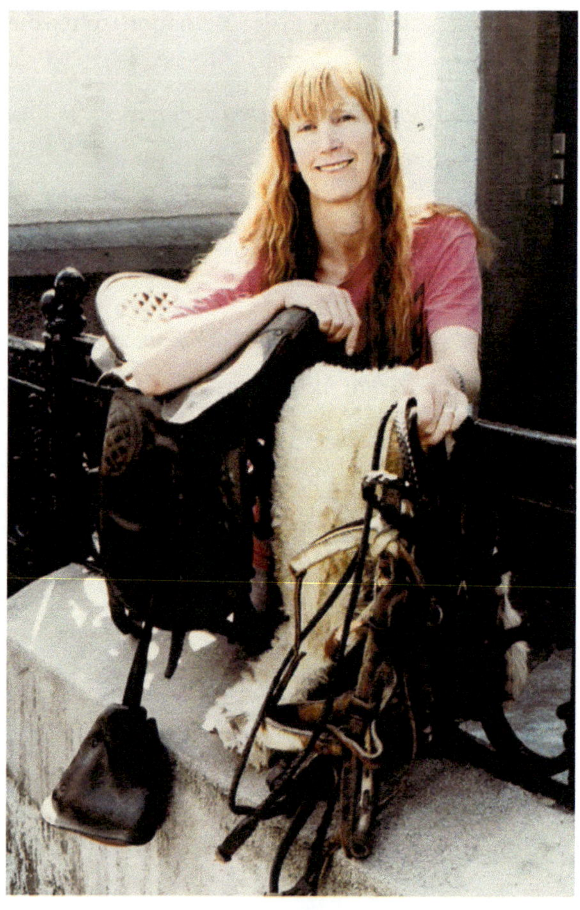

Rosie, at home in Wales, with her saddle, tack and sheepskin chaps used on her incredible journey.
Image © author

CHAPTER TEN

WIM HOF

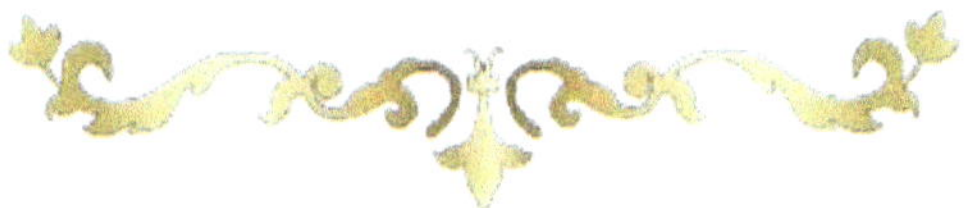

THE ICEMAN

(b.1959)

"If you learn how to use your mind, anything is possible." Wim Hoff

Surely, by now, everyone has heard of The Iceman? With a nick-name like that it demands some curious attention. I mean, surely he can't defeat the cold? What about hypothermia and its resulting affects? Well, he is not the only one practising control of one's body temperature, among other things, and benefitting from it. Though it's likely true that Wim is the first person to actually seek out snow and ice and spend so much time in it.

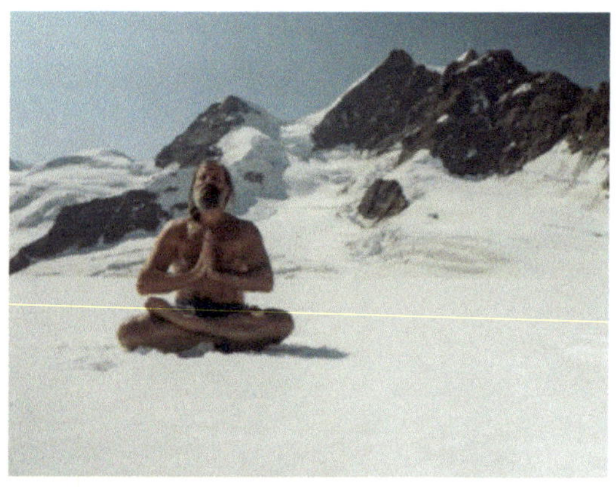

Wim Hoff. Probably safe to say he is not praying!
More likely his breathing technique.
Permission from Leila Zafar B2B - Events - Media Requests

The Naga Sadhus of India and the Himalayas are labelled as the most ascetic of any humans. They endure the most difficult and trying circumstances involving leaving behind all worldly attachments — all those things usually thought of as basic requirements for living. To become a Naga Sadhu is an intense period of tests that can take 10 and sometimes 20 or even 30 years to complete. Imagine spending the rest of your life never sitting or lying down, but always on your feet. Some do this.

All adherents must undergo deep pain and tiresome processes to test their self-control, like folding one leg for years or holding a hand high in the air for years.

We react to such practices as stupid and pointless without realising that these acts, these incredible feats of endurance—and pain, are raising their level of consciousness to the highest level. They learn to transcend pain, and the mostly prosaic, repetitious routines of everyday life. When a Naga Sadhu looks at one of us lesser mortals, he can judge our level of consciousness and psyche in a glance.

An interesting historical record exists about the British colonisation of India. Most colonisation processes involve destruction or dismantling of the culture and traditions of a country. Britain met with and tried to destroy what they saw as a weird and strange way of living. They arranged and instructed a group of Muslim spies—Indian soldiers called sepoys, working for the British government. The sepoys were instructed to keep a close watch on the Nagas and report their movements. The trouble was, after observing them in one place, they were unable to locate them again. This happened so often that eventually the British ended the operation, describing it as the uppermost mystery of India.

The Nagas may eat only once a day, if that. Some choose to live in places that us ordinary people would regard as too wet or cold or isolated or all of these. However, many of them choose to live among people in the warmer climes of India. Some Naga

Sadhus, then, do have a connection with Wim Hof in terms of accepting the cold. The Naga Sadhus don't sleep on beds or mattresses. They sleep on the ground and at most, may use a cloth to lie on. Most are naked or wear a single piece of cloth draped over them. They have overcome the need to feel warmth and comfort. Wim is maybe not at their extreme level, or maybe he is! Who am I to judge that?

As a European, he has, unusually, discovered that control of one's body temperature is possible, among other body systems—control previously thought uncontrollable. And his great tests of endurance should be acknowledged for previously being believed impossible—until he did them!

I first saw Wim Hof on a television documentary a few years ago. I saw him sitting on an iceberg, cross-legged, wearing only a pair of shorts. It grabs your attention for being so out of the normal. He got up and dived into the sea and swam leisurely towards another iceberg. I was immediately intrigued and wanted to know more.

I learnt he had 4 small children and that his wife had mental health problems that doctors weren't able to satisfactorily fix and one day she took her life. Wim found it very hard to deal with—who wouldn't?

One winter's morning, he walked to a quiet place to think things out and suddenly felt impulsed to go in the lake. He stripped off and broke the thin ice and slowly went in and under. He described the calm and quiet moments before emerging and noticed he was not feeling cold. I'm sure some of the finer details have been lost in translation, as they say, but it wasn't the last time he did this by any means. Nor the first.

At the age of 17 he was walking along a frozen canal in an Amsterdam park and suddenly felt the urge to jump in. He stripped off and did just that. He tells of noticing how his mind fell silent. So that was the first step towards becoming the Iceman. He says that while in the icy water of the canal, he barely noticed the cold and felt a different state of awareness in himself. He said it gave him a high for the rest of the day.

From the first publicity came a series of challenges from the media to continue the keen public attention on something so new and different. The challenges led to him breaking 26 Guinness Book of Records. Some of these have since been beaten, but I'm guessing Wim is the first person to have so many records to his name. Some of them are:

- Swimming underneath ice for 66 metres (some reports say 50 metres). This was almost a disaster because he swam without goggles and his eyeballs froze making him unable to see the hole in the ice he was supposed to swim to. A quick-thinking assistant pulled him out in the nick of time.
- Completing a marathon across the Namib Desert in temperatures up to 40C without any drinks.
- Running a full marathon in the Arctic circle, with temperatures to -20C, barefoot, wearing only shorts.

• Climbing 22,000ft up Mt Everest wearing only shoes and a pair of shorts.

• This one is not, I think a Guinness Record, though maybe it is. He hung by one finger on a bar fastened between two hot-air balloons at an altitude of 2000 metres.

David Blaine, an American illusionist, endurance artist, and extreme performer, once stayed inside a block of ice for 55 hours (according to him that was the number of hours, speaking on the Joe Rogan Show) while other reports had it at 58 and 66 hours. How does that stunt compare with Wim? David Blaine wore a woollen hat, a light shirt, trousers and boots and the air he breathed was through entry and exit tubes. The outside air temperature was quite warm, so the air he was breathing was warmer than being out on an iceberg like Wim. One of David Blaine's spokesmen confirmed it was warm inside the ice because of the piped air temperature. So it turns out to be a case of comparing apples with oranges.

In many TV chat shows Wim has told how he was ridiculed and laughed at for 30 years, called crazy and irresponsible. Yet all that publicity eventually attracted scientific minds to wondering just how he seemed to defy the limits of human physiology. Some scientists even told him what he was doing was physiologically impossible. Another way, I guess, of disbelieving what he appeared to be doing.

Since the beginnings of medical science it has been steadfastly believed—assumed is a better word in view of what has been learned through Wim—that the autonomic nervous system and the immune system are systems that work in the background without any input from our consciousness.

When Wim told scientists he could control his body temperature and influence his autonomic nervous system and immune system, they smiled at his apparent naivety and belief in something they knew was not possible. When he was covered in electrodes and immersed in ice up to his neck for well over an hour (112 minutes), the scientists were astounded that his monitored skin temperature was not showing the expected drop they assumed was inevitable.

They ended up telling Wim that he must be a freak of nature because this was not possible. He told them he had a twin brother. That caused some consternation because scientists get excited when a person they are monitoring has a twin. Wim also challenged the scientists by offering to teach a dozen people previously not involved in what he does. He asked them to give him a couple of weeks and they would be able to do the same. This was done and the scientists had to admit that not only was Wim not a freak of nature but that the long held understandings about how human physiology works was about to be re-written.

Splendidly, American school text-books about human physiology are already being re-written. Hopefully the rest of the world will follow suit.

Why is this important? Wim describes how he suffered from deep depression after losing his wife and claims his cold therapy is what fixed him and gave him back a happy, healthy life. He claims that his method can cure PTSD, anxiety, fear and trauma—all conditions of which are difficult or seemingly impossible to treat effectively by medical doctors and specialists. Those conditions are more widespread around the world than ever before and something is needed to reverse this direction. Of course there is scepticism about how his method can cure the list of things he talks about. But scepticism is a healthy thing initially, provided you have an open mind. And Wim's method is increasingly being taken up and practiced.

One example of Wim's belief in his method being proved by science was a 2014 study by Dr. Matthijs Kox and physician Peter Pickkers at Radboud University Medical Centre in the Netherlands. They injected 2 dozen healthy people with an endotoxin that causes chills, headaches and fevers. The ones trained by Wim were unaffected by the toxin while the others succumbed. The doctors believed it was the breathing technique Wim taught which had allowed the deliberate secretion of adrenaline to stop inflammation by the toxin. This was the first scientific proof that humans can control their own immune system through a taught skill. Wim's discoveries are not the only hard-to-believe things some humans can do. They are not as common in the western world as they are in India and the Himalayan countries.

Decades ago NASA scientists put an Indian yogi into a space capsule in their laboratories. They could monitor his physiological status while inside. He demonstrated he could rely on less oxygen than was thought of as necessary, and, slow down his heart beat. At one point he actually stopped his heart and caused panic with the scientists. No doubt, all those years ago, this man was taken to be a freak of nature too. Wim has also shown science that he can control the rate of his heart beat.

Wim's willingness to teach others how to benefit from the cold like he has done, is teaching what he terms his three steps or pillars: Breathing, Cold Therapy, and Commitment.

Breathing is fundamental to life, as we all know, but how you breath is rarely given much thought. Most people, it seems, let breathing happen the way it just seems to happen. There is no conscious effort to change what appears to be an autonomous system that is assumed to know how to work without being interfered with by any conscious thinking.

A recent bestselling book called *'Breath'* by James Nestor tells of some remarkable facts that we ignore at our peril. If you value your health, you have to learn to breath. James Nestor had been a mouth breather all his life till he realised he was seriously compromising his health.

Like the long-held scientific belief that we can't control our temperature and immune systems etc it was also believed that bone formation went downhill after about the age of 30. In the words of one of James Nestor's dentists, Dr Theodore Belfor, the conventional science of bone loss is bullshit. He says anyone can continue to grow bone even well into old age.

I highly recommend reading James Nestor's book, as does Wim Hof, who's name is prominent on the front cover, endorsing it.

So what is this **First Pillar of Breathing**? Look at YouTube and search for Wim Hof and there are so many to choose from. They lead you through a routine which for beginners may start at 3 rounds of 30 breaths, with an increasing breath hold at each round's completion starting at 30 sec and by the end of the third round is one and a half minutes. Some have slow breaths and some have fast breaths. For me, the slow breaths somehow enabled me to hold my breath at the end of each round more easily than fast rounds to the point of comfortably holding for 3-5 minutes on the last round.

If you click through the videos you will see increasingly higher numbers. If you don't attend a local Wim Hof Centre it becomes a case of trial and error till you find what's comfortable, though increasing the number of rounds and breath-holding times will benefit you more. Recently I have seen 10 rounds, with breath holds up to 5 minutes for the last round. Something to work towards though for now 4 rounds seems enough, though clearly not for beginners!

The **Second Pillar** is **Cold Therapy**. This usually starts with cold showers. It can, though not necessarily, move onto ice baths and climbing snow covered mountains in boots and shorts. Some even go to cryotherapy sessions where they go into a small chamber with cold air at temperatures -90C to -120C.

Unsurprisingly, one stays inside for only 2-4 minutes. This is not universally available and can be expensive.

The benefits of cold therapy require frequent exposure. A one-off will not change you, but it will surprise you as to how good you feel. Some of the listed benefits are speeding up metabolism, reducing inflammation, reducing swelling and relieving aching muscles. It is being linked to an improved quality of sleep, higher energy levels, an improved immune system and better mental focus.

Wim's **Third Pillar** is **Commitment**.[1] I like that, because commitment is surely a necessity in any productive way of living. Wim says that by committing oneself to the breathing and cold therapies, you will increase your willpower. Why is that important? Well, the soft, molly-coddled lives modern living seems to prefer, where we are always in a warm place with clothes that are chosen to keep that feeling of warmth and comfort a constant feature, is actually doing us a disservice. Our skin, our largest organ, is crammed full of temperature sensors that without stimulation will atrophy, and like any unused muscles, become flabby and weak without any physical work or exercise. Having a sudden cold shower, or jumping into icy water or having an ice bath will waken up those sensors, stimulating them into action.

As Wim has said in some of those TV chat shows, *"The cold is my friend."*

So how has Wim Hof influenced me? His Iceman activities in the snow, ice and freezing water impressed me tremendously and made me think about it all for months. I read up more about his methods and made a conscious effort to at least start the breathing exercise and cold showers.

For the record, I have, for over a year, had a cold shower every morning. After waking up, I do the breathing session[3], then go straight into the cold shower for at least 5 minutes. Then, without drying myself, I clean my teeth, have a wet shave with water and soap, and 5 minutes of eye exercises. That can take up to 20 minutes not including the breathing exercise. By then, I hardly need a towel as I am almost dry anyway. That is when I get dressed. So far, I have only had three ice baths at home. Again, there was no shivering. Who'd have thought that was possible? Of course, Wim Hof and his devotees would have no problem with that and now, neither do I.

***

There are Wim Hof Centres for teaching the three pillars springing up all over the world. Some people even travel from far away places to Wim Hof's Centre in Europe. An example of an Australian one is, *"Leah Scott's Health Retreats & Wim Hof Instructor,"* based in the Snowy Mountains[2]. As the photos show, she engages a lot of people in cold therapy and other health-promoting activities.

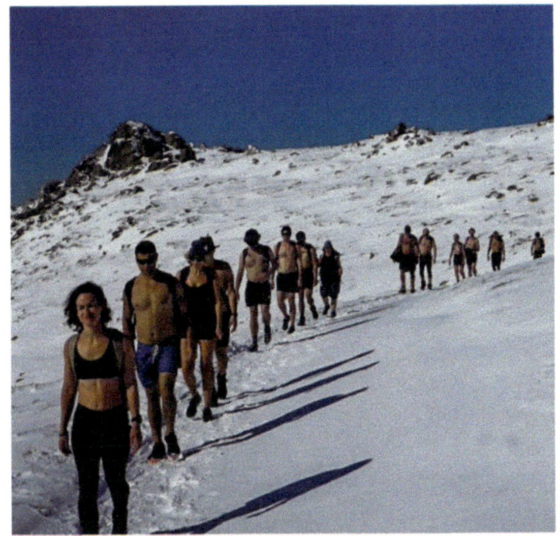

A walk in the Snowy Mountains in winter.
Image courtesy Leah Scott, Wild Things

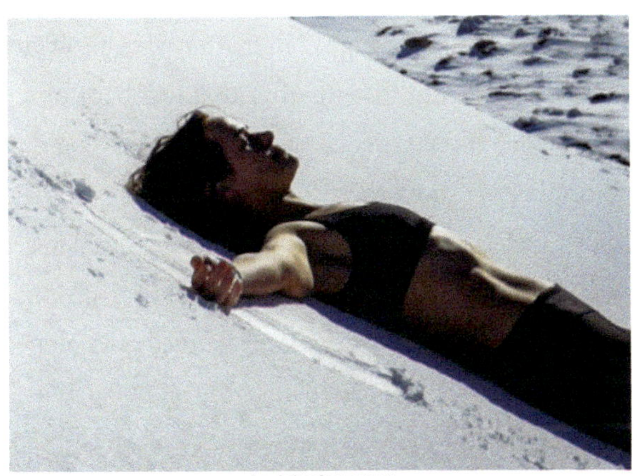

Leah having a rest.
Image courtesy Leah Scott, Wild Things

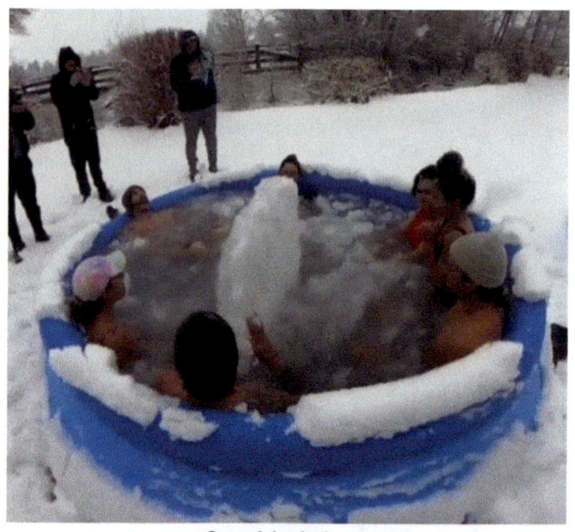

Open air ice-bath
Image courtesy Leah Scott, Wild Things

Do I feel healthier? Yes. Do I feel more energy? Definitely. And I'll add another benefit Wim has often talked of. Going into the cold gives you a high. No matter what problems you might be dealing with, seconds after that first blast of icy cold water hits you, all extraneous thoughts vanish. I've even felt myself smiling as I stand there in cold water. On another Wim Hof video I watched recently, Wim was being interviewed. He was asked what the breathing exercise did for people. Wim replied that it was another example of assumed physiology 'gone west'! Brain scans show which part of the brain is active during different things going on. A patient's brain scan may show a diseased area. Scans light up different parts of the brain. After doing Wim's breathing technique,100% of the brain lights up! Doctors were amazed.

I thank Wim Hof for changing my life for the better. I hope one day to meet him. Wim's infectious humour and enthusiasm shows what a positive and happy person he is.

There is a hard-to-forget very funny moment he shared with a bunch of people who joined him in a trek up a snow covered mountain in Europe. They climbed almost to the top, to the boundary between the two countries. Unknown to them, some soldiers from the neighbouring country were arriving on the other side of the final ridge, dressed in all their full-on winter equipment. As they reached the top and looked down, they couldn't believe what they were seeing. A group of people wearing only boots and shorts. They were astonished and went down to meet them. After a few minutes they were all laughing and taking selfies of each other.

See! Another benefit of Cold Therapy! It improves cross-cultural relations!

REFERENCES/LINKS

[1] *The Wim Hof Method*

[2] *Leah Scott, Wild Things Anatomy*

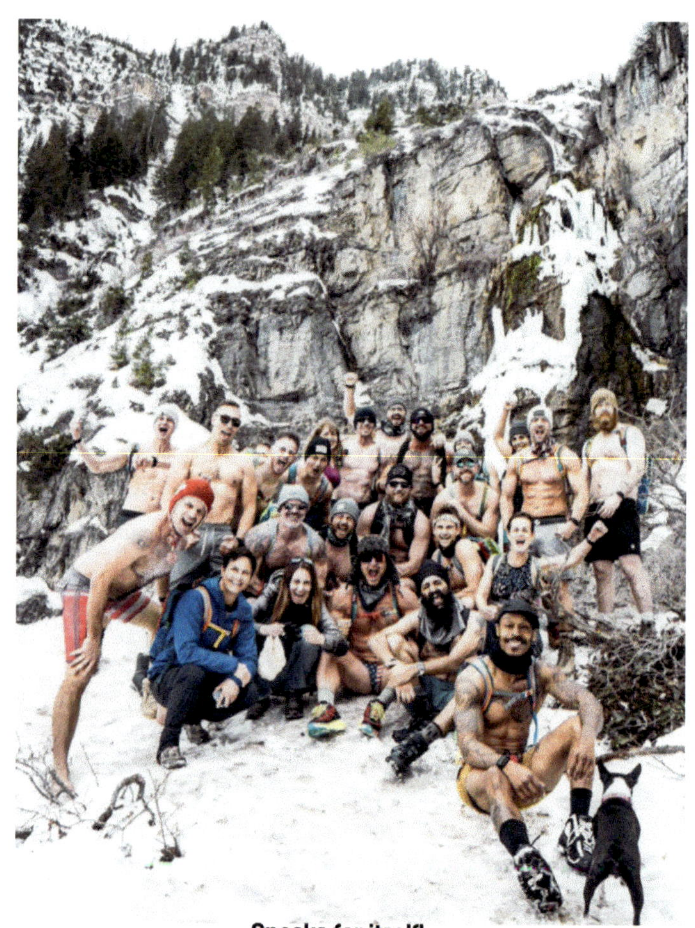

Speaks for itself!
Image courtesy Leah Scott, Wild Things

Epilogue

To all these special people ...

- Your qualities make you stand out from the crowd
- You dared to be different
- I'll never forget your deep influence
- Once met, never forgotten

How did these **'10 Indelibles'** change my life? In many ways, though briefly and mainly, as follows;

Swein Macdonald proved to me beyond doubt that some people have an ability to not only see things from afar, but also to somehow see into the future, even in minute detail. Like Ingo Swann, Alois Irlmaier and Edgar Cayce, they aren't always a 100% successful, but mind-blowing when they are.

John Tonkin made me realise that one's eyesight is not destined to fade with age. Thanks to him I do not need glasses and don't expect to ever need them.

Don Greenbank somehow fixed my damaged spine in 5 minutes after all medical interventions failed over a period of one and a half years. Without Don, my life would not have allowed me to do all the things I have done, including heavy building in stone, mountain trekking while carrying a heavy pack, and much travelling.

Major-General Charles George Gordon lived long before my time. I greatly admire his sense of social justice for those living in places where human rights didn't exist, where life was a free-for-all and slavery was common. I learned from him to not live under a fear of imagined or possible threat of any kind, which in today's world causes much anxiety and stress. I also admire his tenacity in persevering against unlikely odds. Like Churchill, a British Bulldog!

Sir Geofroy Tory removed all doubts for me about the power of dowsing. I need no scientists to try and dissuade me that it works after meeting him. He also demonstrated dowsing is not just about finding water.

John Rodley taught me valuable life skills about how to be an unaffected person—unaffected by all those social conventions that seem only to create bland and uninteresting 'citizens'.

Alexander Selkirk AKA Robinson Crusoe, gave me a permanent sense of dealing with seemingly impossible odds. OK, I haven't been tested to the extent Selkirk was, though, like General Gordon, I am never ready to give in. A neighbour calls me a bulldog, for that same reason.

Daniel Bruhin W, my good friend in Chile, has substantially increased my knowledge of Selkirk and the Juan Fernandez archipelago to my great satisfaction. His persistence in thorough research for, and the very high quality of, his published books has filled a potential void of losing significant records of maritime history of the South Seas in a format available and appreciated by the public everywhere.

Alan Brown, my uncle, taught me the value of keeping high principles in the face of corruption. In the early part of his career, he stuck his neck out many times at the risk of losing his job while being ostracised by co-workers and even management. In later years soccer clubs sought him out to be their coach for his thoroughness and innovative tactics that became the norm in soccer everywhere. He was sought as a manager because of his reputation for fixing corruption.

Rosie Swale-Pope has changed my life by extending my perception of endurance to a far higher level. In a different way to Wim Hof, she continually demonstrates not giving in or giving up when prudence would say otherwise. She has the highest level of 'guts' of any person I have ever met.

Wim Hof has given me the gift of influencing the cells of my body to behave and react as nature intended, with untold health benefits assured. He also re-affirmed my mistrust of medical science and advice. I venture an opinion that Wim might not agree with— that he has 'invented' a new concept: Asceticism is now possible on a part-time basis, allowing continuance of life we know, mixed with cold showers and ice baths that stimulate our senses and provide big health benefits.

To the Reader

I hope you enjoyed this book. If you did, please leave a review — a quick and easy way to support the work of independent authors like me. Thank you.

The author's other non-fiction books, for all the family, can be seen on his webpage: *selkirk4books.com*

About the Author

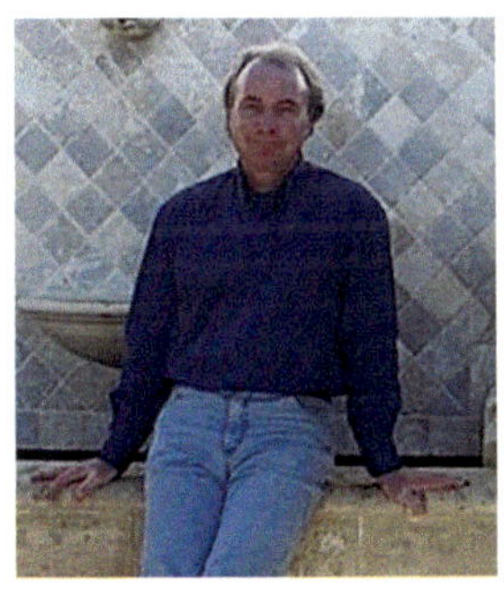

P.A. Brown authors a variety of non-fiction books from air travel hacks, to people with extraordinary abilities, to scary but true stories, how-to's and notebooks and password keepers.

His interests, even from a young age, include ancient stonework and the oddities and curiosities of the world — especially the unexplained. This causes much travel —

twice around the world, foot-slogging in remote places in many countries and islands. He has a high interest in good environmental practice.

The image below is the author camping in winter at 11000' (3353 metres) on Mt Erciyes in Central Turkey.

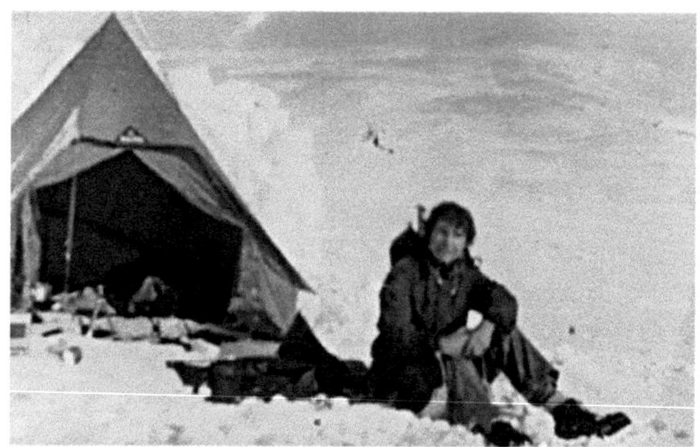

ND - #0139 - 080726 - C45 - 203/127/9 - PB - 9780646864600 - Gloss Lamination